D0344451

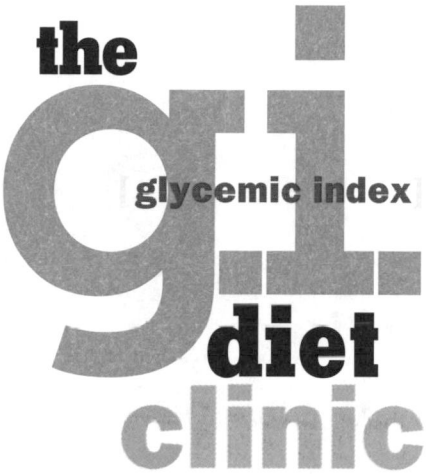
the
g.i.
glycemic index
diet
clinic

Contents

Introduction vii

Part One: The G.I. Diet

chapter one: | **The Truth about Carbs, Fats, and Protein** 2

chapter two: | **The Secret to Easy, Permanent Weight Loss** 10

chapter three: | **The G.I. Diet Essentials** 15

chapter four: | **Before You Start** 39

chapter five: | **The G.I. Diet Clinic Pantry** 46

Part Two: The Thirteen-Week G.I. Diet Clinic

| **Week 1: Getting Started** 50

| **Week 2: Meal Planning** 63

| **Week 3: Behavior Change** 73

| **Week 4: Falling Off the Wagon** 85

| **Week 5: Eating Out** 93

| **Week 6: Unrealistic Expectations** 109

| **Week 7: Emotional Eating** 117

| **Week 8: Reaching a Plateau** 129

| **Week 9: Staying Motivated** 137

| **Week 10: Your Health—What's at Stake** 149

| **Week 11: Holidays, Celebrations, and Special Events** 159

| **Week 12: Exercise** 169

| **Week 13: When Weight Loss Causes Anxiety** 183

| **Beyond Week 13: Phase II** 193

Part Three: The Recipes

| **Breakfast** 202
| **Soups** 211
| **Salads** 215
| **Meatless** 227
| **Fish and Seafood** 237
| **Poultry** 245
| **Meat** 257
| **Snacks** 264
| **Desserts** 272

Part Four: Appendixes

appendix 1: | **Results of the e-Clinic** 284
appendix 2: | **The Complete G.I. Diet Food Guide** 290

Indexes

| **General Index** 303
| **Recipe Index** 315

Introduction

Ever since I wrote the original *G.I. Diet* back in 2002, my mission has been to help as many people as possible lose weight and keep it off. It all began during my own personal struggle to lose weight. Though I had been working to raise awareness of heart disease and stroke as president of the Heart and Stroke Foundation of Ontario and was earnestly promoting healthy lifestyle choices among Canadians to reduce their risk for those diseases, the sad truth was that I was overweight myself. In an effort to lose the extra pounds, I tried deprivation diet after starvation diet, weighed everything I put into my mouth, and calculated calories, points, and carbohydrates. But nothing I tried worked; I could never manage to lose more than a few pounds. It was so frustrating and demoralizing that if I hadn't felt duty-bound as the chief representative of the foundation to walk the walk, I may well have given up. But I knew how dangerous my habits were to my health, and I doggedly persevered.

When I eventually started a diet based on the principles of the glycemic index (G.I., which measures the speed at which your body breaks down carbohydrates and converts them to glucose, the vehicle your body uses for energy), I miraculously lost the extra weight that had been plaguing me for so long. I realized that while I'd been blaming myself and my lack of willpower, the real reason I hadn't been able to slim down was that I didn't have the right information.

During my search for an effective diet, the two main problems I encountered were first, that I often felt as if I were going hungry or being deprived, and second, that I was frustrated by the difficulty of having to track calories, points, formulas, and ratios. I was confident that if I could find a way of eating that eliminated these two fundamental problems, I could help people lose weight and improve their health.

The result was the G.I. Diet, a nutritionally ideal way to eat that emphasizes low-glycemic-index foods such as fruits and vegetables, whole grains, low-fat dairy products, as well as lean protein and the "best" fats. As you will see, unlike many other diets, the G.I. Diet doesn't eliminate any food groups. Its easy-to-follow color-coded system means you will never have to count calories or points, or weigh or measure food. You won't go hungry or feel deprived. It will keep you feeling satisfied and energetic as you slim down to your ideal weight.

THE ORIGINS OF THE E-CLINIC

Since the original *G.I. Diet* book hit the shelves, I've heard from tens of thousands of people who are thrilled with their weight loss on the program. The Diet proved so successful that word quickly spread, and to date over two million copies have been sold in eighteen languages in twenty-three countries.

But as well as hearing about successes, I also heard a lot about readers' challenges and frustrations. Most of these individuals were coming to the G.I. Diet after a long string of other attempts to manage their weight; they had tried every diet under the sun and had still failed time and time again. There were clearly some issues people were struggling with that needed to be addressed directly—the loss of confidence and the low self-esteem that came with the repeated failure of earlier diets had certainly had an effect. Food was a comfort, giving these individuals a short-term feeling of well-being, but as the numbers on the scale climbed higher, it was also a curse. Clearly, many dieters needed help and encouragement—not to get them on track (they were great at starting out), but to help them stay there.

I faced a dilemma. My books are, by their nature, a monologue or a one-way communication: I discuss the diet, tell the readers what to do, and that's it—end of the book. But what these chronic dieters needed was not a monologue—they needed a dialogue. With this in mind, I set out to develop a way of building an interactive experience with G.I. Diet participants, where we could communicate with each other in real time as they were actually going through the very process of trying to lose weight.

This effort resulted in a thirteen-week e-Clinic that I conducted through my website, www.gidiet.com. The volunteer participants were all of above-average weight and had struggled with their weight for most of their lives. I hypothesized that if I could help these "hard" cases to successfully shed excess pounds, then I could certainly help those with more modest weight challenges.

The concept was simple: Start with the already user-friendly G.I. Diet, and make it even *more* user-friendly by leading participants in detail through the first thirteen critical weeks. During this time, they would be coached on the components of the program: how to handle crises such as falling off the wagon or getting stuck on a plateau, and most important, how to stay motivated—even in the face of unexpected weight gain or cravings for fattening foods. In addition, we would share our day-to-day challenges and discuss solutions as a group. This would be conducted by way of weekly communication: I would send the group a newsletter addressing a particular concern commonly faced by G.I. dieters, as well as the full weekly menu and shopping list. In return, once a week each participant would send me his or her weight and measurements and a weekly diary illustrating any questions or concerns encountered over the course of the clinic. I would then review and highlight some of the issues raised in their diaries and incorporate them into the following week's electronic newsletter.

Though hundreds of people applied for the e-Clinic, I could choose only thirty-five to participate. Remarkably, of those thirty-five, over 80 percent stuck with the e-Clinic until the very end (and those who dropped out did so for unrelated health problems). By the end of the thirteen weeks, the average weight loss per person was an incredible 25 pounds—and perhaps more amazing, an average loss of 10 inches from the waist and hips. As for me, I received a wealth of feedback that I knew would be tremendously helpful to others trying to achieve their weight-loss goals.

This book is a faithful reproduction of the e-Clinic that I conducted with those thirty-five people on the G.I. Diet. You'll share the same experiences they did: the same menus, the same advice, most likely the same kinds of highs and lows, and—ultimately—the same success.

HOW TO USE THIS BOOK

In **Part One,** I explain the principles of health and nutrition, the basics of successful weight loss, and how the G.I. Diet works. It's not complicated at all: You'll get a list of foods to include (green-light), those to avoid (red-light), and foods to eat when you achieve your target weight (yellow-light—proceed with caution), and information on how to make sensible decisions when shopping, cooking, or reading a food label.

Because a knowledge of nutrition and the mechanics of weight loss are critical to your success, I recommend you read this section closely before moving on and refer back to it over the course of the Clinic. With a complete understanding of what exactly is happening in your body, you will greatly enhance the value of the Clinic and thus greatly enhance your chances of success. Don't worry—this isn't a college-level science class. This is everyday information that's sensible and easy-to-follow.

Part Two is the heart of the book—the thirteen-week Clinic program broken down into week-by-week chapters. Each one deals with a different core aspect of success on the G.I. Diet—matters such as behavior change, staying motivated, and the temptation that leads to falling off the wagon. My discussion of each topic is accompanied by what the participants in the original e-Clinic had to say about these subjects, along with my responses.

The weekly sequence is laid out in an intentional order that typically corresponds to the experiences you'll have over the course of three months on the G.I. Diet. Week 1, for instance, is "Getting Started," while Week 8 is "Reaching a Plateau"—a frequent concern by the second month of any diet. The Clinic, however, is not rigid! If you find yourself stuck on a weight plateau during the fifth or tenth week, reread or fast-forward to the appropriate chapter. Of particular note is Week 11, "Holidays, Celebrations, and Special Events," which addresses those times when we often find it difficult to stick to our healthy eating habits. Of course, visit the advice and recommendations for this week when a holiday or celebration comes up on your calendar—move it up a few weeks, or push it back, as you need it.

Each week also includes a detailed meal plan (three daily meals, plus snacks), along with an accompanying grocery list for the week's meals. These plans are both optional and flexible, depending on your personal preferences. Although some people who prefer a fully structured program might follow each day to the letter, others might prefer to plan their own green-light meals and snacks, using the meal plan only as a guide.

● **Green-light foods:** *Eat as much as you like.*

● **Yellow-light foods:** *Eat only when you have achieved your target weight.*

● **Red-light foods:** *Avoid entirely.*

For more information, see page 13.

There's also diary space for you to record your measurements as well as observations of or comments on your weekly experience with the diet and your changing lifestyle.

Once you've concluded your thirteen weeks, the next chapter deals with life post-Clinic. You'll read e-Clinic participants' closing thoughts after their experiences, and—for when you reach your own target weight—you'll learn about Phase II of the G.I. Diet. In Phase II, we reintroduce some yellow-light treats, and modify your diet to prevent both losing and gaining any additional weight so you can maintain your new healthy weight for the rest of your life.

When I ran the original e-Clinic, the participants requested an extension to the program, and so for the next nine months the majority of the group and I did monthly e-mail check-ins—rounding their experience out to a full year. Once you've made it through the thirteen weeks outlined in this book, you are invited to sign on for a further nine monthly e-mail letters that will provide you with support, the latest news on green-light products and dishes, as well as more recipes and tips. I also invite you to submit your own monthly diary and measurements in response to these letters—an ongoing e-Clinic of your very own! See page 198 for more information on this program.

Part Three lists more than sixty delicious recipes broken down by meal type—virtually all the recipes you'll need in order to make the dishes suggested in each week's meal plan. The recipes are green-light, low-G.I., and (best of all) delicious—you'll know you've made the right choice of diet when you try the recipe for Pecan Brownies!

The recipes are followed by **Part Four,** which consists of two appendixes. The first gives the results achieved by some of our e-Clinic participants and includes their thoughts on the program. The second is a comprehensive breakdown of common foods and ingredients, categorizing the contents into the three traffic light colors—red, yellow, and green. It's a handy reference for times when your palate wanders away from the meals and recipes indicated elsewhere in the book.

A NEW WAY OF EATING

Whether this is your first introduction to the G.I. Diet program or you're an old hand looking for a new approach, I'm confident that this Clinic will help you lose weight permanently. It's not so much a diet as it is a new way of eating—one that allows you to lose weight without going hungry or feeling deprived. The traffic light color-coding of foods keeps it simple, so you'll never have to count another calorie again. Not only that, but it's a balanced, nutritious diet that will help you to reduce your risk of major diseases and to live a longer, healthier, and more active life.

the g.i. diet clinic

glycemic index

A 13-Week Plan for Permanent and Healthy Weight Loss

RICK GALLOP

workman publishing ■ new york

To the original e-Clinic members, whose commitment, enthusiasm, and honesty over the course of the twelve-month program made this book possible.

Copyright © 2008 by Green Light Foods Inc.

All rights reserved. No portion of this book may be reproduced—mechanically, electronically, or by any other means, including photocopying—without written permission of the publisher.

Library of Congress Cataloging-in-Publication Data is available.

ISBN 978-0-7611-4948-4

Cover design by Barbara Balch
Book design by Robb Allen and Netta Rabin

Workman books are available at special discounts when purchased in bulk for premiums and sales promotions as well as for fund-raising or educational use. Special editions or book excerpts can also be created to specification. For details, contact the Special Sales Director at the address below.

Workman Publishing Company, Inc.
225 Varick Street
New York, NY 10014-4381

www.workman.com

Printed in the United States of America

First printing October 2008
10 9 8 7 6 5 4 3 2 1

Part One

The G.I. Diet

chapter one:

The Truth About Carbs, Fats, and Protein

IT'S JUST ABOUT IMPOSSIBLE TO LIVE IN THIS COUNTRY AND NOT know that we are in the midst of an "obesity epidemic." If you watch television, listen to the radio, read the newspaper, or simply glance over the magazine headlines at the supermarket checkout, you can't help but be aware that nearly two thirds of Americans are overweight, with half of those categorized as clinically obese.

Everyone seems to have an explanation for our collective weight crisis: Some hold the fast-food industry responsible, others blame our sedentary lifestyle. Some maintain we are eating too much fat, others say we are eating too many carbohydrates. So what's the truth?

Well, all of these reasons are part of the answer, but it's a far less complex matter than many would have us believe. If you reduce the problem to its physiological cause, it's actually quite simple: We're consuming more calories than we're expending, and the resulting surplus is stored around our waists, hips, and thighs as fat. There's no mystery here.

Expending calories is a matter of exercise (see page 169 for my tips on that), but the G.I. Diet isn't about the calories we expend, it's about the calories we take in. There's no need here to obsessively count or track your calorie consumption—I've said it in each and every one of my G.I. Diet books, and I'll say it again now: The key to healthy, sustainable weight loss is a true understanding of nutrition. To understand why we are consuming more calories, and to understand how that is leading to our growing waistlines, we need to get back to basics and look at the three fundamental elements of our diet: carbohydrates, fats, and protein. We need to understand the roles these components play in the digestive system and how they work together—whether we're in the process of getting fat or thin.

CARBOHYDRATES

We'll start with carbohydrates, a hot topic with a bad rap ever since the popularity of low-carbohydrate diets like the Atkins program has catapulted them to national attention. Carbohydrates have been so much in the news over the past few years that we refer to them in shorthand—"carbs"—to save a few syllables. Though carbs are often blamed for all our weight problems, their role in weight control has really been misunderstood. The foods we refer to as carbohydrates, such as bread, grains, potatoes, and other starches, are a necessary part of a healthy diet. They are rich in fiber, vitamins, and minerals, and include antioxidants, which we now know play an important role in the prevention of heart disease and cancer. The primary source of energy for our bodies, carbohydrates are found not only in breads and starches, but also in vegetables, fruits, legumes (beans), and dairy products.

Here is how carbs work: When you eat an orange or a bagel, your body digests the carbohydrate compounds in the food and turns them into glucose, a type of sugar that is easily convertible to energy. The glucose dissolves in your bloodstream and then travels to the parts of your body that use energy, such as your muscles and brain. When managing weight, however, it is important to realize that not all carbs are created equal.

Some carbohydrate-laden foods break down into glucose in the digestive system at a slow and steady rate, gradually releasing their nutrients and keeping us feeling full and satisfied. Others break down rapidly, spiking our glucose levels and then dissipating quickly, leaving us feeling hungry again. For example, cornflakes and old-fashioned oatmeal are both carbohydrates, but we all know the difference between eating a bowl of oatmeal for breakfast and eating a bowl of cornflakes. The oatmeal stays with you—it "sticks to your ribs," as my mother used to say—whereas an hour after eating the cornflakes, your stomach starts rumbling again, pushing you toward your next snack or meal. Throughout the course of a day, if you are eating the sorts of carbs that break down rapidly, as opposed to those that break down slowly, you will be eating more and, as a result, will begin to put on weight. If, however, you start eating carbs that break down slowly, like old-fashioned rolled oats, you will eat less and begin to lose weight.

Selecting the right type of carbohydrate is key to achieving your optimum energy and weight. But how do you know which carbohydrate is the right type and which isn't? Well, the first clue is the amount of processing the food has undergone. The more a food is processed beyond its natural, fibrous state, the less processing your body has to do to digest it. The quicker you digest the food, the sooner you feel hungry again. This helps explain why the number of adults who are overweight has surged over the past sixty years. A hundred years ago, most of the food people ate came straight from the farm to the dinner table. Lack of refrigeration and scant knowledge of food chemistry meant that most food remained in its original state until it hit the home kitchen, and the vast majority of foods' nutrients and fiber were preserved, helping slow the breakdown of glucose in our bloodstreams. Advances in food science and processing technology in the 1940s and '50s, however, led to a revolution in prepared foods geared to speeding up and simplifying mealtimes. The giant food companies—Kraft, Kellogg, Del Monte, Nestlé, and others—were born, as were the first fast-food restaurants. We happily began spending more money for the convenience of prepared, processed, packaged, canned, frozen, and bottled food. The fast-food era had begun.

It was during this period that the miller's traditional wind and water mills were replaced with high-speed steel rolling mills that stripped away the bran, fiber, and wheat germ, which could spoil, and produced a talcum-like powder: today's white flour. This fine white flour has the benefit of textural consistency and a longer shelf life, but it is also devoid of those nutrients and components that help regulate the breakdown of glucose. White flour is the basic ingredient for most of our breads and cereals, as well as for baked goods and snacks such as cookies, muffins, crackers, and pretzels. Walk through any supermarket and you will be surrounded by towering stacks of these flour-based processed products. We're eating more and more of these foods: Over the past three decades, our consumption of grain has increased by 50 percent. And our bodies are paying the price for this change.

The second clue in determining whether a carbohydrate is the right type is the amount of fiber it contains. Fiber, in simple terms, provides low-calorie filler. It does double duty, in fact: It literally fills up your stomach, so you feel satiated; and your body takes much longer to break it down, so it stays with you longer and slows the digestive process. There are two forms of fiber: soluble and insoluble. Soluble fiber is found in carbs such as oatmeal, beans, barley, and citrus fruits and has been shown to lower blood cholesterol levels. Insoluble fiber is important for normal bowel function and is typically found in whole wheat breads and cereals, and most vegetables.

There are two other important components that inhibit the rapid breakdown of food in our digestive system, and they are fats and protein. Let's look at fats first.

FATS

Fat, like fiber, acts as a brake in the digestive process. When combined with other foods, fat becomes a barrier to digestive juices. It also signals the brain that you are satisfied and don't require more food. Does this mean that we should eat all the fat we want? Definitely not!

Though fat is essential for a nutritious diet, because it contains various key elements that are crucial to digestion, cell development, and overall health, it also contains twice the number of calories per gram as carbohydrates and protein. If you decide to "just add peanut butter" (which can be low-carb and high in protein) to your otherwise disciplined regime, it doesn't take much of it—two tablespoons—to spike your total count by almost 200 calories.

Also, your body is a genius at hanging on to fat and refusing to let it go. This is because fat is how the body stores reserve supplies of energy, usually around the waist, hips, and thighs. Fat is money in the bank as far as the body is concerned—a rainy-day investment for when you have to call up extra energy. This clever system originally helped our ancestors survive during periods of famine. The problem today is that we don't live with cycles of feast and famine—it's more like feast and then feast again! But the body's desire for fat continues, along with its reluctance to give it up.

This is why losing weight is so difficult: Your body does everything it can to persuade you to eat more fat. How? Fat makes things taste good. Juicy steaks, chocolate cake, and rich ice cream taste better than a bean sprout. That's the fat content talking.

Sorry to say, there's no getting around it: If you want to lose weight, you have to watch your fat consumption. In addition, you need to be concerned about the type of fats you eat because many are harmful to your health.

There are four types of fat: the best, the good, the bad, and the really ugly. The "really ugly" fats are potentially the most dangerous, and they lurk in many of our most popular snack foods. They are vegetable oils that have been heat-treated to make them thicken—the trans fats you've been hearing so much about in the media lately. They raise the amount of LDL, or bad, cholesterol in our bodies while lowering the amount of HDL, or good, cholesterol, which protects us from heart disease. As a result they boost our cholesterol levels, which thickens our arteries and causes heart attack and stroke. So avoid using trans fats, such as vegetable shortening and hard margarine, and avoid packaged snack foods, baked goods, crackers, and cereals that contain them. (You can spot them by checking labels for "hydrogenated" or "partially hydrogenated" oils.)

The "bad" fats are called saturated fats, and they are for the most part solid at room temperature (think of butter, cheese, or the fat found on an uncooked steak). While saturated fats almost always come from animal sources, there are a couple of others you should be aware of, too: Coconut oil and palm oil are two vegetable oils that are saturated and, because they are cheap, are used in many snack foods, especially cookies. Saturated fats directly elevate your risk of heart and Alzheimer's diseases. The evidence is also growing that many cancers, including colon, prostate, and breast cancer, are associated with diets that are excessively high in saturated fats.

The "good" and "best" fats are both unsaturated, and those fall into two categories. The good fats are called polyunsaturated, and they are cholesterol free. Most vegetable oils, such as corn and sunflower, are good fats. What you really should be eating, however, are the best fats, monounsaturated, which actually promote good health. These are the fats found in olives, almonds, and canola and olive oils. Monounsaturated fats have a beneficial effect on cholesterol and are good for your heart. This is one reason the incidence of heart disease is low in Mediterranean countries, where olive oil is a staple. Although fancy olive oil is expensive, you can enjoy the same health benefits from less costly supermarket brands.

Another highly beneficial oil that falls into the "best" category is omega-3, a fatty acid found in deep-sea fish, such as salmon, mackerel, albacore tuna, and herring, as well as in lake trout, walnuts, and flaxseed and canola oils. Some brands of eggs and liquid eggs also contain omega-3, which can help lower cholesterol and protect cardiovascular health—look for it advertised on the packaging.

So the "best" and "good" fats are an important part of a healthy diet and also help slow digestion. Still, they're fats and they pack a lot of calories. We have to be careful, then, to limit our intake of poly- and monounsaturated fats when trying to lose weight.

Since protein also acts as a brake in the digestive process, let's look at it in more detail.

PROTEIN

Protein is an absolutely essential part of your diet. In fact, you are already half protein: 50 percent of your dry body weight is made up of muscles, organs, skin, and hair, all forms of protein. We need this element to build and repair body tissue, and it figures in nearly all metabolic reactions. Protein is also a critical brain food, providing amino acids for the neurotransmitters that relay messages to the brain. This is why it's not a good idea to skip breakfast on the morning of a big meeting or exam. The "brain fog" people experience on some diets is likely the result of diminished protein. Protein is literally food for thought.

The main sources of dietary protein come from animals: meat, seafood, dairy, and eggs. Vegetable sources include beans and soy-based products such as tofu. Unfortunately, protein sources such as red meat and full-fat dairy products are also high in "bad" saturated fats, which are harmful to your health. It is important that we get our protein from sources that are low in saturated fats, such as lean meats, skinless poultry, seafood, low-fat dairy products, cholesterol-reduced liquid eggs, and tofu and other soy products.

One exceptionally good source of protein is the humble bean. Beans are a perfect food, really: They're high in protein and fiber, and low in saturated fat. No wonder so many of the world's cuisines have found myriad wonderful ways to cook beans. I truly believe that North Americans need to become more bean savvy. Along similar lines, nuts are another excellent source of protein and are relatively low in fat—as long as you don't eat a whole bowlful.

Protein is much more effective than carbohydrates or fat at satisfying hunger. It will make you feel fuller longer, which is why you should try to incorporate some protein into every meal and snack. This will help keep you on the ball and feeling satisfied.

Now that we know how carbohydrates, fats, and protein work in the digestive system, let's use the information to discover how to take off the extra pounds.

TO SUM UP

- Eat carbohydrates that have not been highly processed and that do not contain highly processed ingredients.
- Eat less fat overall and look for low-fat alternatives to your current food choices.
- Eat only monounsaturated and polyunsaturated fats.
- Include some protein in all your meals and snacks.
- Eat only low-fat protein, preferably from both animal and vegetable sources.

chapter two:

The Secret to Easy, Permanent Weight Loss

THE "G.I." IN G.I. DIET STANDS FOR *GLYCEMIC INDEX*, WHICH IS the basis of this way of eating—and the only scientific phrase you'll need to know. The glycemic index is the secret to reducing calories and losing weight without going hungry. It measures the speed at which carbohydrates break down in our digestive system and turn into glucose, the body's main source of energy or fuel (see page 3 for a refresher on how this works).

The glycemic index was developed by Dr. David Jenkins, a professor of nutritional sciences at the University of Toronto, when he was researching the impact of different carbohydrates on the blood sugar, or glucose, level of diabetics. He found that certain carbohydrates broke down quickly and flooded the bloodstream with sugar, but others broke down more slowly, only marginally increasing blood sugar levels. The faster a food breaks down, the higher its rating on the glycemic index, which sets pure sugar at 100 and scores all other foods against that number. These findings were important to diabetics, who could then use the index to identify low-G.I., slow-release foods that would help control their blood sugar levels. In general, foods with a G.I. of above 60 can be considered high-G.I, and those with a G.I. of below 50 are low-G.I. Below are some examples of the G.I. ratings for a single serving of a range of popular foods.

EXAMPLES OF G.I. RATINGS

High G.I.	Low G.I.
Baguette 95	Orange 44
Cornflakes 84	All-Bran 43
Rice cake 82	Oatmeal 42
Doughnut 76	White-flour spaghetti 41
Bagel 72	Apple 38
Cereal bar 72	Beans 31
Cookie 69	Plain yogurt 25

What do these G.I. ratings have to do with the numbers on your bathroom scale? Well, it turns out that low-G.I., slow-release foods have a significant impact on our ability to lose weight. As I have explained, when we eat the wrong type of carbohydrate—i.e., a high-G.I. food—the body quickly digests it and releases a flood of sugar (glucose) into the bloodstream. This gives us a short-term high, but the sugar is just as quickly absorbed by the body, leaving us with a post-sugar slump. We feel lethargic and start looking for our next sugar fix. A fast-food lunch of a double cheeseburger, fries, and a Coke delivers a short-term burst of energy, but by midafternoon we start feeling tired, sluggish, and hungry. That's when we reach for "just one" brownie or bag of potato chips. These high-G.I. foods deliver the rush we want and then quickly drop us down again. The roller-coaster ride is a hard cycle to break. But a high-G.I. diet will make you feel hungry more often, so you end up eating more and gaining more weight.

Let's look at the other end of the G.I. index. Low-G.I. foods—such as fresh fruits and vegetables, whole grains, pasta, beans, and low-fat dairy products—take longer to digest, deliver a steady supply of sugar to our bloodstream, and leave us feeling fuller for a longer time. Consequently, we eat less. It also helps that these foods are generally lower in calories than their high-G.I. counterparts are. As a result, we consume less food and fewer calories without going hungry or feeling unsatisfied.

The key player in this process of energy storage and retrieval is insulin, a hormone secreted by the pancreas. Insulin does two things very well. First, it regulates the amount of sugar (glucose) in our bloodstream, removing the excess and storing it as glycogen for immediate use by our muscles or putting it into storage as fat. Second, insulin acts as a security guard at the fat gates, reluctantly giving up its reserves. This evolutionary feature is a throwback to the days when our ancestors were hunter-gatherers, habitually experiencing times of feast or famine. When food was in abundance, the body stored its surplus as fat to tide it over the inevitable days of famine.

Of course, food is now readily available to us at the nearest twenty-four-hour supermarket. But our bodies still function very much as they did in the earliest days. When we eat a high-G.I. food, our pancreas releases insulin to reduce the glucose level in our blood, which, if left unchecked, would lead to hyperglycemia (high blood sugar). If we aren't using all that energy at the moment, the glucose is stored as fat. Soon we become hungry again. Our body can either draw on our reserves of fat and laboriously convert them back to sugar, or it can look for more food. Since giving up extra fat is the body's last choice—who knows when that supply might come in handy!—it would rather send us to the fridge than work to convert fat back to sugar. This helped our survival back in the old days, but it gets in the way of weight loss now.

So our goal is to limit the amount of insulin in our systems by avoiding high-G.I. foods, which stimulate its production, and instead choosing low-G.I. foods, which keep the supply of sugar in our bloodstream consistent. Slow-release, low-G.I. carbohydrates help curb your appetite by leaving you feeling fuller for a longer period of time. When you combine them with lean protein and the best fats, which help slow the digestive process, you have the magic combination that will allow you to lose weight without going hungry.

Determining the G.I. of a particular food is, as it happens, quite complex. But before you begin to worry that I'm breaking my promise of an easy weight-loss plan, check out pages 290–300. These lists of foods, sorted into red, yellow, and green categories, are the Complete G.I. Diet Food Guide. I've done all the calculations, measurements, and math for you, and have sorted the foods you like to eat into one of three categories, based on the colors of the traffic light. Here's how the color-coded categories work:

Red-Light Foods: The foods in the red column are to be avoided. They are high-G.I., higher-calorie foods that will make it impossible for you to lose weight.

Yellow-Light Foods: The foods in the yellow column are mid-range G.I. foods that should be treated with caution. They should be avoided when you are trying to lose weight, but once you've slimmed down to your ideal weight, you can begin to enjoy yellow-light foods from time to time.

Green-Light Foods: The green column lists foods that are low G.I., low in fat, and lower in calories. These are the foods that will allow you to lose weight. Don't expect them to be tasteless and boring! There are many delicious and satisfying choices that will make you feel as though you aren't even on a diet.

If you're a veteran of the low-carbohydrate craze, you'll be surprised to find potatoes and rice in the green-light column—

they are fine as long as they are the right type. Baked potatoes and French fries have a high G.I., but boiled new potatoes have a low G.I. The short-grain, glutinous white rice served in Chinese and Thai restaurants is high G.I., whereas long-grain, brown, basmati, and wild rice are low. Pasta is also a green-light food—as long as it is cooked only until al dente (with some firmness to the bite). Any processing of food, including cooking, increases a food's G.I. because heat breaks down starch capsules and fiber, giving your digestive juices a head start. This is why you should never overcook vegetables; instead, steam them or boil them in a small amount of water just until they are tender. This way, they will retain their vitamins and other nutrients, and their G.I. rating will remain low.

Translated into real food, what does this mean? Well, for dinner you could have a grilled chicken breast, boiled new potatoes, a side salad of romaine lettuce and red pepper dressed with a bit of olive oil and lemon juice, and some asparagus if you feel like it. The trick is to stick with foods that have a low G.I., are low in fat, and are lowish in calories. Although eating green-light foods is really the core of the G.I. Diet, there are a few more things you'll need to know to follow the program, and I discuss these in the next chapter.

TO SUM UP

- Low-G.I. foods take longer to digest, so you feel satiated longer.
- The key to losing weight is to eat low-G.I., low-calorie foods—in other words, foods from the green-light column of the Complete G.I. Diet Food Guide.

chapter three:

The G.I. Diet Essentials

THE G.I. DIET CONSISTS OF THREE PHASES. THE FIRST TWO, the Preliminary Phase and Phase I, are the dramatic parts of the G.I. Diet—the period when those unwanted pounds come off! During these stages, you'll focus on eating foods that are low G.I. and also low in fat and sugar—the foods in the green-light column of the Complete G.I. Diet Food Guide on pages 290–300. Yes, this means a farewell to bagels and a fond adieu to Häagen-Dazs. But it doesn't mean you won't have a multitude of delicious foods to choose from. Once you've reached your ideal weight, you enter Phase II, the maintenance phase of the program, which is the way you will eat for as long as you'd like to stay at your new size.

Depending on how much weight you're setting out to lose, you'll need to determine whether to start with the Preliminary Phase (see page 18) or to skip ahead to Phase I. This determination relies on your body mass index (BMI), which is a measurement of how much body fat you are carrying relative to your height.

YOUR BMI

You can determine your BMI using the table on the next page. Find your height in the left-hand column, and drag your finger to the right until you see the number closest to your current weight. The number at the top of that column is your BMI.

BODY MASS INDEX (BMI)

	normal						overweight					obese		
BMI	**19**	**20**	**21**	**22**	**23**	**24**	**25**	**26**	**27**	**28**	**29**	**30**	**31**	**32**
height (inches)	**body weight (pounds)**													
4'10"	91	96	100	105	110	115	119	124	129	134	138	143	148	153
4'11"	94	99	104	109	114	119	124	128	133	138	143	148	153	158
5'0"	97	102	107	112	118	123	128	133	138	143	148	153	158	163
5'1"	100	106	111	116	122	127	132	137	143	148	153	158	164	169
5'2"	104	109	115	120	126	131	136	142	147	153	158	164	169	175
5'3"	107	113	118	124	130	135	141	146	152	158	163	169	175	180
5'4"	110	116	122	128	134	140	145	151	157	163	169	174	180	186
5'5"	114	120	126	132	138	144	150	156	162	168	174	180	186	192
5'6"	118	124	130	136	142	148	155	161	167	173	179	186	192	198
5'7"	121	127	134	140	146	153	159	166	172	178	185	191	198	204
5'8"	125	131	138	144	151	158	164	171	177	184	190	197	203	210
5'9"	128	135	142	149	155	162	169	176	182	189	196	203	209	216
5'10"	132	139	146	153	160	167	174	181	188	195	202	209	216	222
5'11"	136	143	150	157	165	172	179	186	193	200	208	215	222	229
6'0"	140	147	154	162	169	177	184	191	199	206	213	221	228	235
6'1"	144	151	159	166	174	182	189	197	204	212	219	227	235	242
6'2"	148	155	163	171	179	186	194	202	210	218	225	233	241	249
6'3"	152	160	168	176	184	192	200	208	216	224	232	240	248	256
6'4"	156	164	172	180	189	197	205	213	221	230	238	246	254	263

Source: National Heart, Lung, and Blood Institute

extremely obese																
33	**34**	**35**	**36**	**37**	**38**	**39**	**40**	**41**	**42**	**43**	**44**	**45**	**46**	**47**	**48**	**49**
158	162	167	172	177	181	186	191	196	201	205	210	215	220	224	229	234
163	168	173	178	183	188	193	198	203	208	212	217	222	227	232	237	242
168	174	179	184	189	194	199	204	209	215	220	225	230	235	240	245	250
174	180	185	190	195	201	206	211	217	222	227	232	238	243	248	254	259
180	186	191	196	202	207	213	218	224	229	235	240	246	251	256	262	267
186	191	197	203	208	214	220	225	231	237	242	248	254	259	265	270	278
192	197	204	209	215	221	227	232	238	244	250	256	262	267	273	279	285
198	204	210	216	222	228	234	240	246	252	258	264	270	276	282	288	294
204	210	216	223	229	235	241	247	253	260	266	272	278	284	291	297	303
211	217	223	230	236	242	249	255	261	268	274	280	287	293	299	306	312
216	223	230	236	243	249	256	262	269	276	282	289	295	302	308	315	322
223	230	236	243	250	257	263	270	277	284	291	297	304	311	318	324	331
229	236	243	250	257	264	271	278	285	292	299	306	313	320	327	334	341
236	243	250	257	265	272	279	286	293	301	308	315	322	329	338	343	351
242	250	258	265	272	279	287	294	302	309	316	324	331	338	346	353	361
250	257	265	272	280	288	295	302	310	318	325	333	340	348	355	363	371
256	264	272	280	287	295	303	311	319	326	334	342	350	358	365	373	381
264	272	279	287	295	303	311	319	327	335	343	351	359	367	375	383	391
271	279	287	295	304	312	320	328	336	344	353	361	369	377	385	394	402

Although the BMI gives a relatively accurate measure of body fat, it applies only to people who are twenty to sixty-five years of age. It isn't valid for children, pregnant or nursing women, the elderly, or heavily muscled athletes. For the rest of us, however, it is the only accepted international standard for weight.

If your BMI falls between 19 and 24, your weight is within the acceptable norm and is considered healthy. Anything between 25 and 29 is considered overweight; if you're 30 or over, you are officially obese. Of course, the BMI chart is not infallible—some exceptions can be made for those who are particularly muscular, for example. But by and large it is an excellent gauge of the healthiness of your body weight.

THE PRELIMINARY PHASE AND PHASE I

To determine whether to begin with the Preliminary Phase or with Phase 1, take a look at the BMI chart. If it's 32 or under, I recommend you begin with Phase 1 of the program. If your BMI is over 32, start with the Preliminary Phase. The Preliminary Phase is, in effect, a "step-in" plan that helps reduce any initial hunger pangs caused by a sudden drop in calories that people with a significant weight problem sometimes experience. The Preliminary Phase lasts as long as your BMI is greater than 32.

The primary difference between the Preliminary Phase and Phase I is in the number of times you will eat each day. In the Preliminary Phase, you should be eating three meals and four snacks every day, and in Phase I, three meals and three snacks every day. The reason I recommend an extra snack in the Preliminary Phase is that someone with a larger body requires more calories just to keep functioning on a daily basis than someone who is lighter. This is also why I suggest larger serving sizes for some green-light foods in the Preliminary Phase than in Phase

I. Although I generally do not restrict quantities of green-light foods—within reason (five heads of cabbage is a bit extreme)—there are a few exceptions, which I outline below. (Except where indicated, a serving size is per meal, not per day.)

If you feel that you can manage without the Preliminary Phase, please feel free to go straight to Phase 1. About half of the original e-Clinic members with a BMI of over 32 elected to do this without experiencing significant difficulty.

Regardless of which phase you begin with, when you weigh yourself each week, recalculate your BMI. If you're beginning with Phase I, this is a straightforward measure of your progress. If you're beginning with the Preliminary Phase, it will let you know when you should adjust your eating habits to those of Phase I (remember, Phase I is for those with a BMI of 32 or below).

What Do I Eat—and How Much?

During the Preliminary Phase and Phase I, you will be sticking to the foods listed in the green-light column of the Complete G.I. Diet Food Guide on pages 290–300. To preview your green-light choices for each meal, turn to pages 22–24, 27–30, and 35–36.

Remember, this is not a starvation diet—far from it. Going hungry is simply not necessary for weight loss; in fact, it's something to be resolutely avoided! Hunger is the absolute death knell for any weight-loss program. If you are hungry for a sustained period of time, your body will feel that it hasn't received enough fuel to meet its needs and will slow the rate at which it burns calories, making it even harder to lose those extra pounds. So never leave your digestive system with nothing to do. If it is busy processing food and steadily supplying energy to your brain, not only will your metabolism keep firing at a steady rate, but you won't be looking for high-calorie snacks. This is why you can, within reason, eat as much green-light food as you want on the G.I. Diet. Serving size does matter with a few foods, however, so take a look at the table on page 20.

GREEN-LIGHT SERVINGS

Green-Light Food	Preliminary Phase (BMI of 33 or More)	Phase I (BMI of 32 or Less)
Crispbreads (with high fiber, e.g., Wasa)	3 crispbreads	2 crispbreads
Green-light breads (which have at least 3 grams of fiber per slice)	2 slices per day	1 slice per day
Green-light cereals	⅔ cup	½ cup
Green-light nuts	12 to 15	8 to 10
Margarine (nonhydrogenated, light)	3 teaspoons	2 teaspoons
Meat, fish, poultry	6 ounces	4 ounces (about the size of a pack of cards)
Olive/canola oil	1½ teaspoons	1 teaspoon
Olives	6 to 8	4 to 5
Pasta	1 cup cooked	¾ cup cooked
Potatoes (new or small, boiled)	4 to 5	2 to 3
Rice (basmati, brown, long-grain)	¾ cup cooked	⅔ cup cooked

Filling Your Plate

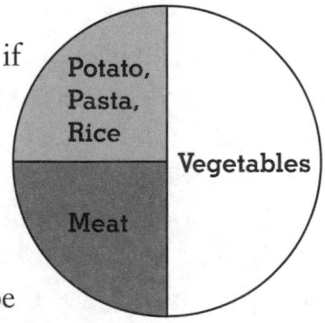

Each meal and snack should contain, if possible, a combination of green-light protein, fats, and carbohydrates (especially those found in fresh vegetables and fruit). An easy way to visualize portion size is to divide your plate into three sections. Half the plate should be filled with vegetables; one quarter should contain protein, such as lean meat, poultry, seafood, eggs, tofu, or legumes; and the last quarter should contain a green-light serving of rice, pasta, or potatoes.

When Do I Eat?

Try to eat regularly throughout the day. If you skimp on breakfast and lunch, you will probably be starving by dinner and end up piling on the food. Have one snack midmorning, another midafternoon, and the last before bed. In the Preliminary Phase, you can eat the fourth snack later in the afternoon if you usually have a late dinner, or during the evening if you generally have an early dinner. It's really up to you—have the extra snack at the time of day you feel you most need it. The idea is to keep your digestive system happily busy so you won't start craving those red-light snacks.

MEAL BASICS

Because the green-light way of eating is most likely new to you, you're probably wondering what to eat instead of that bagel with cream cheese for breakfast, that hamburger for lunch, and those tortilla chips and salsa for a snack. On the following pages I'll go over your various green-light options for each of the main meals and snacks of your daily G.I. program. Let's start with breakfast.

Breakfast

I know you've been told that breakfast is the most important meal of the day, and it's true. It's the first thing you eat after your night-long "fast" of twelve hours or more, and it launches you into your workday. Eating a healthy breakfast will help you avoid the need to grab a coffee and Danish as soon as you hit the office and will make you feel satisfied and energetic. Eating breakfast every day doesn't mean you have to set the alarm any earlier. If you have time to read the paper or feed the cat, you have time to prepare and eat a green-light breakfast.

The following table lists typical breakfast foods in the color-coded categories. To ensure you have a balanced breakfast, include some green-light carbohydrates, protein, and fat. For a complete list of foods, see the Complete G.I. Diet Food Guide on pages 290–300.

Let's take a closer look at some of the usual breakfast choices.

PROTEIN			
meat and eggs	Regular bacon Sausages Whole regular eggs	Turkey bacon Whole omega-3 eggs	Canadian bacon Lean ham Liquid eggs/ egg whites
dairy	Cheese Cottage cheese (whole or 2%) Cream Milk (whole or 2%) Sour Cream Yogurt (whole or 2%)	Cream cheese (light) Milk (1%) Sour cream (light) Yogurt (low-fat with sugar)	Buttermilk (skim/1%) Cottage/cream cheese or sour cream (1% or fat-free) Extra-low-fat cheese Fruit yogurt (fat-free with sweetener) Milk (skim) Soy milk (plain, low-fat)

CARBOHYDRATES			
cereals	All cold cereals except those listed as yellow- and green-light Granola Muesli (commercial)	Kashi Golean Crunch! Kashi Good Friends Shredded Wheat 'N Bran	High-fiber/ low-fat cereals (such as All-Bran Bran Buds and Kashi Golean) Oat bran Oatmeal (old-fashioned rolled oats)

breads/ grains	Bagels Baguettes Cookies Doughnuts Muffins Pancakes/waffles White bread	Crispbreads Whole-grain breads (less than 3g fiber/slice)	100% stone-ground whole wheat bread* Green-light muffins (see pp. 264–268) High-fiber crispbreads such as Wasa Fiber* Whole-grain, high-fiber breads (3g fiber/slice)*
fruits	Applesauce containing sugar Canned fruit in syrup Melons Most dried fruit	Apricots (fresh) Apricots (dried)** Bananas Fruit cocktail in juice Kiwis Mangoes Papayas Pineapples	Apples Berries Cherries Fruit spreads (no sugar added) Grapefruit Grapes Oranges Peaches Plums
juices	Fruit drinks Prune juice Sweetened juices (including "naturally sweetened") Watermelon juice	Apple juice (unsweetened) Grapefruit juice (unsweetened) Orange juice (unsweetened) Pear juice (unsweetened)	Eat the fruit rather than drink its juice
vegetables	French fries Hash browns/ home fries		Most vegetables

*Limit serving size (see page 20).

**Use sparingly.

FATS			
	Butter Hard margarine Peanut butter (regular and light) Tropical oils (such as palm and coconut) Vegetable shortening	Most nuts Natural nut butters Peanut butter (100% peanuts) Soft margarine (nonhydrogenated) Vegetable oils	Almonds* Canola oil* Hazelnuts* Light or low-fat soft margarine (nonhydrogenated)* Olive oil* Pistachios*

*Limit serving size (see page 20).

Coffee and Tea

Okay, this is a tough one. The trouble with coffee is caffeine. It's not a health problem in itself, but it does stimulate the production of insulin. That's part of the "buzz" we get from coffee. But insulin reduces your blood sugar level, which then increases your appetite. Have you ever ordered a latte from Starbucks and then felt positively shaky an hour later? That's your blood sugar hitting bottom. You cure it by eating a bagel—which isn't helpful when you're trying to lose weight. So in Phase I, try to cut out caffeine altogether by switching to decaf. As unpleasant as it may be, caffeine withdrawal will end in time. It's easiest if you cut down gradually: Go from a medium coffee to a small; then try a half-caffeinated, half-decaf blend. Finally limit yourself to decaffeinated coffee—some brands taste as good as the real thing.

If you absolutely must have your caffeine fix, switch to tea. It has only about one third the caffeine that coffee has, and black tea and green tea have health benefits as well: They're rich in antioxidants and beneficial for heart health and reducing the risk of dementia. Green tea is also considered an anticarcinogen. Herbal teas, such as peppermint, chamomile, and other blends, are fine too, as long as they contain no caffeine. If no coffee is going to be a deal breaker, then go ahead, have one cup a day—but not a double espresso. If you take milk and sugar, make it skim milk and a sweetener such as Splenda.

Cereals

Another toughie. Most cold cereals contain hidden or not-so-hidden sugars and are therefore red-light. Green-light cereals are high in fiber; they have at least 10 grams per serving. Admittedly, they're not a lot of fun by themselves, but you can liven them up with the addition of fruit (fresh or frozen is best, but canned will do), a few nuts, or some fruit yogurt (fat-free, with sugar substitute).

My personal favorite cereal is good old-fashioned oatmeal—not the instant type that comes in packets, but the slow-cooking rolled oats kind—and it's catching on. They're even starting to serve it in high-end hotels now! This kind of oatmeal is not only low G.I., but also low calorie and has been shown to lower cholesterol. Yes, you have to cook it, but it takes only about three minutes or so in the microwave, and not much longer for one portion on the stovetop. Dress it up with yogurt, sliced almonds, berries, or unsweetened applesauce. It's also just fine with nothing but milk on it. I probably receive more e-mails about people's delight at rediscovering oatmeal than about any other food or meal. Give it a try.

Toast

Go ahead with your breakfast toast, but have no more than one slice per meal. Also, make sure your bread has at least 3 grams of fiber per slice. (Note: Some bread labels quote a two-slice serving, which should equal 6 grams per serving.) The best choice is 100% stone-ground whole wheat bread, which has a coarser grind and therefore a lower G.I. Keep away from white bread, cracked wheat, and anything else made with white flour—they're red-light.

Butter and Jams

Butter is out. It's very high in saturated fat, and despite the protestations of the dairy industry, it's not good for your health or waistline. Yes, it does make things taste good—that's what fat does best. But you can still enjoy any one of a variety of light, nonhydrogenated soft margarines—if you use only a teaspoon or so. When buying fruit spreads, look for the "extra fruit/no sugar added" varieties. Fruit, not sugar, should be the first ingredient listed. These varieties taste great and don't have the calories of the usual commercial jams.

Dairy

Low-fat dairy products are an ideal green-light choice and an excellent source of protein. I have a glass of skim milk every morning, though I admit that skim didn't taste great at first. But I weaned myself off 2 percent by switching to 1 percent before moving on to skim. Now 2 percent tastes like cream!

Fat-free yogurt with sugar substitute instead of sugar is ideal for breakfast, dessert, or a snack, either by itself or added to fruits or cereals. Low-fat cottage cheese is also a top-rated green-light source of protein. Or you can make a low-fat soft cheese spread by letting yogurt drain in cheesecloth overnight in the refrigerator.

Regular full-fat dairy products, including whole milk, cream, cheese, and butter, are loaded with saturated fat and should be avoided completely.

Eggs

Use liquid eggs, which are sold near the whole eggs at the supermarket and come in what looks like a milk carton. They are lower in saturated fat and cholesterol than regular eggs, and they make wonderful omelets. Otherwise, separate whole eggs and eat only the whites. If you're eating a hotel or restaurant breakfast, in most cases the kitchen is happy to make omelets with egg whites only.

Bacon

Bacon is red-light because of its high saturated-fat content. There are tasty green-light alternatives, however—such as Canadian bacon and lean ham—that make great BLTs or sides for your eggs.

Lunch and Dinner

Lunch and dinner offer us a plethora of meal choices, from healthy salads to fat- and calorie-laden steaks and creamy pastas. Eating green-light is a simple matter of planning ahead: Choose recipes and ingredients that are green-light, and take a moment to enjoy the act of cooking your dinner or packing your brown-bag lunch. For a more specific take on lunch and dinner, look at each meal's breakdown on the following pages (Lunch is on page 30, and Dinner begins on page 31). Use the guidelines here for making your selections, and for a complete list of foods, see the Complete G.I. Diet Food Guide on pages 290–300.

PROTEIN			
meat, eggs, poultry, fish	Breaded fish and seafood Fish canned in oil Ground beef (more than 10% fat) Hamburgers Hot dogs Pâté Processed meats Regular bacon Sausages Sushi Whole regular eggs	Chicken legs, thighs, and wings (skinless) Ground beef (lean, 6–10% fat) Lamb (lean cuts) Pork (lean cuts) Tofu Turkey bacon Whole omega-3 eggs	All fish and seafood (not breaded or canned in oil) Beef (lean cuts) Chicken breast (skinless) Ground beef (extra lean—95% fat-free or more) Lean deli meats Liquid eggs and egg whites Pork tenderloin Soft tofu (low-fat) Turkey breast (skinless) TVP Veal

(continued)

PROTEIN *(CONTINUED)*			
dairy	Butter Cheese Cottage cheese (whole or 2%) Milk (whole or 2%) Sour cream Yogurt (whole or 2%)	Cheese (low-fat) Milk (1%) Sour cream (light) Yogurt (low-fat)	Cheese (fat-free) Cottage cheese/ sour cream (1% or fat-free) Fruit yogurt (fat-free with sweetener) Milk (skim) Soy milk (low-fat)

CARBOHYDRATES			
breads/ grains	Bagels Baguettes and other crusty white breads Biscuits Cake and cookies Croissants and pastries Croutons Hamburger/hot dog buns Muffins/doughnuts Noodles (canned or instant) Pasta filled with cheese or meat Pizza Rice (short-grain, white, instant) Tortillas White sandwich bread and other non-whole-grain sandwich bread	Crispbreads with fiber Pita (whole wheat) Tortillas (whole wheat) Whole-grain breads	100% stone-ground whole wheat bread* High-fiber crispbreads* Pasta (any shape, preferably whole-wheat), cooked al dente* Quinoa and other whole grains Rice (basmati, brown, long-grain)* Whole-grain, high-fiber breads (3g fiber per slice)*

*Limit serving size (see page 20).

fruits/ vegetables	Fava beans French fries Melons Most dried fruit Parsnips Potatoes (mashed or baked) Rutabagas	Apricot (fresh) Apricots (dried)** Bananas Beets Corn Kiwis Mangoes Papayas Pineapples Pomegranates Potatoes (boiled) Squash Sweet potatoes Yams	Apples Arugula Asparagus Avocado (¼) Beans (green/wax) Bell peppers Blackberries Broccoli Brussels sprouts Cabbage Carrots Cauliflower Celery Cherries Cucumbers Eggplant Grapefruit Grapes Hot peppers Leeks Lemons Lettuce Mushrooms New or small potatoes (boiled) Olives* Onions Oranges Peaches Pears Peas Pickles Plums Radishes Raspberries Snow peas Spinach Strawberries Tomatoes Zucchini

*Limit serving size (see page 20).

**Use sparingly.

FATS			
	Bottled salad dressings (regular) Butter Hard margarine Mayonnaise Peanut butter (regular, light) Tropical oils (such as palm and coconut) Vegetable shortening	Bottled salad dressings (light) Corn oil Mayonnaise (light) Most nuts Peanut butter (no sugar added) Soft margarine (nonhydrogenated) Vegetable oils Walnuts	Almonds* Canola oil* Hazelnuts* Mayonnaise (fat-free) Olive oil* Pistachios* Salad dressings (low-fat, low-sugar) Soft margarine (nonhydrogenated, light)* Vinaigrette

SOUPS			
	All cream-based soups Canned black bean Canned green pea Canned pureed vegetable Canned split pea	Canned chicken noodle Canned lentil Canned tomato	Chunky bean and vegetable soups (e.g., Campbell's Healthy Request, Healthy Choice) Homemade soups with green-light ingredients

*Limit serving size (see page 20).

Lunch

Lunch is usually the most problematic meal for dieters because we tend to eat it outside the home and in a hurry. Taking your lunch to work is the easiest way to ensure you eat green-light. And there are other advantages to brown-bagging it, besides avoiding the temptation of a red-light lunch: It's cheaper, and it gives you downtime at your desk to read or catch up on paperwork. The ground rules for brown-bagging lunch can be found on the Lunch and Dinner table on page 27–30. For a complete list of foods, see the Complete G.I. Diet Food Guide on pages 290–300

Sandwiches

Sandwiches are a lunchtime staple, and it's no wonder: They're portable and easy to make, and they offer endless variety. They can also be a dietary disaster, but if you follow the suggestions below, you can keep your sandwiches green-light.

- Always use 100 percent stone-ground whole wheat or high-fiber whole-grain bread (3 grams of fiber per slice).
- Sandwiches should be served open-faced. Either pack components separately and assemble just before eating or make your sandwich with a "lettuce lining" that helps keep the bread from getting soggy.
- Include at least three vegetables, such as lettuce, tomato, red or green bell pepper, cucumber, sprouts, or onion.
- Instead of spreading the bread with mayonnaise, butter, or margarine, use mustard or hummus.
- Add up to 4 ounces of cooked lean meat or fish: roast beef, turkey, shrimp, or salmon.
- If you make tuna or chicken salad, use low-fat mayonnaise or low-fat salad dressing and celery.
- Mix canned salmon with malt vinegar or fresh lemon.

Salads

Preparing salads may seem more labor-intensive than making sandwiches, but it doesn't have to be. Invest in a variety of reusable plastic containers so you can take individual-size salads to work. Keep a supply of green-light vinaigrette (see pages 215–216) on hand, and wash greens ahead of time and store in paper towels in plastic bags. You'll find that salads are a creative way to use up leftovers with a minimum of fuss.

Dinner

Dinner is traditionally the main meal of the day. We usually have more time for eating at the end of the day, and we generally feel fatigued as well, which encourages us to consume more. But because we will probably be spending the evening relaxing rather than being active before going to bed, it is important that we don't overdo it. For dinner guidelines, see the Lunch and Dinner table on pages 27–30. For a complete list of foods, see the Complete G.I. Diet Food Guide on pages 290–300.

No dinner is complete without protein. But the portion size is not without limits: Whether it is in the form of meat, poultry, seafood, beans, or tofu, it should cover no more than one quarter of your plate. A serving size should be 4 ounces,* which is roughly the size of the palm of your hand.

Red Meat

Though most red meat does contain saturated fat, there are ways to minimize it:

- Buy only low-fat cuts of beef, such as top round. For making hamburgers or spaghetti sauces, buy extra-lean ground beef. Veal and pork tenderloin are low in fat, too. As for juicy steaks, well, they are juicy because of the fat in them, so they're not a good choice.
- Trim any visible fat from the meat. Even a quarter inch of fat can double the total amount of fat grams you consume.
- Broiling or grilling allows the excess fat from the meat to drain off. (Try one of the George Foreman–style fat-draining electric grills.)
- For stovetop cooking, use a little vegetable oil spray rather than oil. The spray goes further.

Poultry

White-meat chicken and turkey breast are excellent green-light choices, provided that the high-fat skin is removed. In the yellow-light category are skinless thighs, wings, and legs, which are higher in fat.

*For Preliminary Phase servings, see page 20.

Seafood

This is always a good green-light choice. Although certain cold-water fish, such as salmon and cod, have a relatively high oil content, this oil is omega-3 and is beneficial to your heart health. Shrimp and squid are fine, too, as long as they aren't breaded or battered. A plate of fish and chips, alas, is out.

Beans and Legumes

If you don't think you're into beans, it's time to reevaluate! Beans are an excellent source of so many good things: fiber, low-fat protein, and "good" carbs that deliver nutrients while taking their time going through the digestive system. And they are a snap to incorporate into salads and soups to up the protein quotient. Chickpeas, lentils, navy beans, black beans, kidney beans—there's a bean for every day of the week. But watch out for canned pork and beans, which is high in sugar and fat, and avoid canned bean soups, which are processed to the point where their overall G.I. rating is too high. Homemade bean soups, however, are an excellent choice. You will find several delicious recipes using beans in the recipe section of this book.

Tofu

You don't have to be a vegetarian to enjoy tofu, which is low in saturated fat and an excellent source of protein. Although tofu is not necessarily flavor-packed on its own, it takes on the flavors of whatever seasonings and sauces it is cooked with. Seasoned tofu scrambles, for instance, are a good substitute for scrambled eggs. Choose soft tofu, which has up to one third less fat than the firm variety.

Textured Vegetable Protein (TVP)

This isn't a new device for prerecording TV shows! TVP, a soy alternative to meat, looks a lot like ground beef and can be used in the same ways—in lasagna, chili, stir-fries, and spaghetti sauce. It's quite tasty and delivers the texture of meat with a fraction of the calories and fat. Our middle son, a vegetarian who has since left the nest, put us on to this adaptable product.

Potatoes, Pasta, Rice

These carbohydrates should cover only one quarter of the plate. Remember, when it comes to potatoes, your first choice is boiled new or small potatoes. Most other choices, especially baked potatoes or French fries, are red-light. Sweet potatoes are a good lower-G.I. food, but since they tend to come in larger sizes, I suggest you save them for Phase II. Your serving of pasta should be no more than ¾ cup cooked—just until al dente. If you have rice, make it ⅔ cup cooked basmati, wild, brown, or long-grain rice.*

Vegetables

Here you can put the measuring cup away. Eat as many vegetables and as much salad as you like; they should be the backbone of your meal. Always include at least two vegetables, and remember to cook them until just crisp-tender. Experiment with something you've never had before. Baby bok choy is delicious grilled, and broccoli rabe, a dark green vegetable that looks like broccoli with more leaves, is a nice change. Dark, curly green vegetables such as kale are full of good things, including folic acid. Greens such as lettuces or baby spinach come conveniently prewashed in bags. Frozen bags of vegetables are also convenient and inexpensive; you can even toss the veggies into a saucepan and add tomato juice with a dollop of salsa for a quick vegetable soup.

Dessert

Yes, dessert is part of the G.I. Diet—at least the kind of dessert that is green-light and good for you. This includes most fruits, as well as low-fat dairy products, such as frozen yogurt and ice cream sweetened with sugar substitute rather than sugar. If you like to

*For Preliminary Phase servings, see page 20.

make your desserts from scratch, see pages 272–281 for some mouthwatering green-light cookies, brownies, and other treats.

Snacks

Keep your digestive system busy and your energy up with between-meal snacks—four a day during the Preliminary Phase and three a day during Phase I. Try to eat balanced snacks that include a bit of protein and carbohydrates, for example a piece of fruit with a few nuts, or cottage cheese with celery sticks.

A convenient snack for when you're on the go is half a nutrition bar. Be careful when choosing one: Most are full of cereal and sugar. The ones to look for have 20 to 30 grams of carbohydrates, 12 to 15 grams of protein, and 5 grams of fat per 50-gram bar.

Keep in mind that many snacks and desserts labeled "low-fat" or "sugar-free" aren't necessarily green-light. Sugar-free instant puddings and low-fat muffins are still high-G.I. because they contain highly processed grains.

DESSERT AND SNACKS			
	Bagels Candy Cookies Crackers Doughnuts Flavored gelatin (all varieties) French fries Ice cream (full-fat) Muffins (except homemade green-light muffins) Popcorn (microwaved or pre-popped)	Bananas Dark chocolate (70% cocoa) Ice cream (low-fat) Most nuts Popcorn (air popped)	Almonds* Applesauce (unsweetened) Canned peaches/pears in juice or water Cottage cheese (1% or fat-free) Extra-low-fat cheese (e.g., Laughing Cow Light, Boursin Light) Fruit yogurt (fat-free with sweetener)

(continued)

*Limit serving size (see page 20).

DESSERT AND SNACKS *(CONTINUED)*			
	Potato chips Pretzels Pudding Raisins Rice cakes Sorbet Tortilla chips Trail mix White bread		Hazelnuts* Homemade green-light snacks (see pp. 264–271) Ice cream (low-fat and no added sugar) Most fresh fruit Most fresh vegetables Nutrition bars** Pickles Pistachios* Pumpkin seeds Sugar-free hard candies Sunflower seeds

*Limited serving size (see page 20).

**180–225 calorie bars, e.g., ZonePerfect or Balance bars; ½ bar per serving.

What Do I Drink?

Because liquids don't trip our satiety mechanisms and fill us up, it's a waste to take in calories through them. Unfortunately, many beverages are high in calories. People often treat regular soft drinks and fruit juices as nonfoods, but this is how extra calories slip by us. Juice, for example, is a processed product—even freshly squeezed—and has a much higher G.I. than whatever fruit or vegetable it is made from. A glass of orange juice contains nearly two and a half times the calories of a fresh orange and none of the fiber! So eat the fruit or vegetable rather than drink its juice. That way you'll get all the benefits of its nutrients and fiber while consuming fewer calories. As well, stay away from any beverage that contains added sugar or caffeine. As I explained earlier, caffeine stimulates insulin, which leads to our feeling hungry. So no coffee or soft drinks containing caffeine in Phase I. That said, fluids are an important part of any diet (I'm sure you're all familiar with the eight-glasses-of-water-a-day prescription). The following are your best green-light choices:

Water

The cheapest, easiest, and best thing to drink is plain water. Seventy percent of our body consists of water, which is needed for digestion, circulation, regulation of body temperature, lubrication of joints, and healthy skin. We can live for weeks without food, but we can survive only a few days without water. Don't feel you have to drink eight glasses of water a day in addition to other beverages. Milk, tea, and soft drinks all contribute to the eight-glass recommendation. But do try to drink a glass of water before each meal—it will help you feel fuller so that you don't overeat.

Skim Milk

After a skeptical start, I've grown to really enjoy skim milk. It has all the protein, calcium, and other vitamins of whole and 2 percent, with a fraction of the calories. I particularly like to drink it with breakfast and lunch, which tend to be a little short on protein. Skim milk is an ideal green-light choice.

Soft Drinks

If you're used to drinking soft drinks, you can still enjoy the sugar- and caffeine-free diet ones. They are available in a wide variety of flavors. For an elegant treat, try some club soda or seltzer with a wedge of lemon or lime.

Tea

Tea is an excellent green-light beverage. Although black and green teas do contain caffeine, the amount is negligible—only about one third that of coffee. And besides tasting delicious, tea has health benefits as well. Black and green teas contain antioxidant properties that help prevent heart and Alzheimer's diseases. In fact, tea has more flavonoids (antioxidants) than any vegetable tested. Two cups of black or green tea have the same amount of antioxidants as 7 cups of orange juice or 28 cups of apple juice.

So tea in moderation is fine—minus the sugar and cream, of course. Try some new varieties: Darjeeling, Earl Grey, English Breakfast or spicy chai (with sugar substitute). Herbal teas, as long as they are caffeine-free, are also a green-light option, though they lack the flavonoids. Iced tea is acceptable if it's sugar-free.

Alcohol

Alcohol is generally a disaster for any weight-loss program. It puts your blood sugar on a roller coaster: You go up and feel great, then come down and feel like having another drink or eating the whole bowl of peanuts. Alcohol also contains lots of calories. So in Phase I, put away the corkscrew. See page 160 for some ideas on how to tide yourself over at a cocktail party or another social event.

Now that you have some basic ideas of what you'll be eating, it's time to get ready to start. In the next chapter, I'll outline the steps for launching yourself into the program.

TO SUM UP:

- In the Preliminary Phase and Phase I, eat only green-light foods.
- Eat three balanced meals plus four snacks a day in the Preliminary Phase and three balanced meals plus three snacks in Phase I.
- Pay attention to portion size: the palm of your hand for protein, and a quarter plate for pasta, potatoes, or rice. Use common sense and eat moderate amounts.
- Drink plenty of fluids, including an 8-ounce glass of water with meals and snacks (but no caffeine or alcohol).

chapter four:

Before You Start

UNFORTUNATELY, MOST PEOPLE VIEW A DIET AS A SHORT-TERM change in eating habits that is ditched once weight-loss targets have been achieved. They then revert to their old dietary habits and, not suprisingly, are soon back at their original weight, or worse. You won't find that here! *The G.I. Diet is not so much a diet as it is a completely new and permanent way of eating.* This is without question the most important message in this book.

The G.I. Diet is an ideal way to eat for the rest of your life. A constant refrain I've heard from the tens of thousands of successful participants is that they have happily made the G.I. Diet way of eating a permanent part of their lives. Your motivation to lose weight is high, and with the G.I. Diet you now have the action plan that will help you make those unwanted pounds disappear. Still, to be successful, you are going to have to make some significant changes in your life. The better prepared you are, the better equipped you will be to handle any challenges that may arise. The following six steps will get you off to the best possible start.

1. Go see your doctor. Before starting any major change in your eating patterns, schedule a general checkup with your doctor or health care practitioner. This serves two purposes: First, it's important to see if you have any unaddressed health issues that could affect your weight-loss plans. And second, having a baseline measurement of your health before starting the Diet will give you a crystal clear picture of just how much your health improves once you are on the road to your target weight! As you lose weight, your overall health will certainly get better, and it will be wonderfully motivating to learn that your blood glucose levels have improved or that your blood pressure has gone down. Along the way, it may even be possible to change medications you might be taking for weight-related conditions such as diabetes or high blood pressure, though that decision should be left to your doctor.

2. Assess whether it's the right time to start. Although you shouldn't use this as an excuse to indefinitely postpone embarking on the Diet, make sure that you're ready to make a major change in your eating habits. Are you in the middle of a job change? A major house renovation or move? Is it the week before Christmas or before the cruise you've been planning for a year? Then it's probably not the best time to completely overhaul your pantry. Some life events will make it harder—or even impossible—for you to give the program the attention it needs or to stick with it. Choose a period when your life is relatively stable and when you have time to learn new eating habits—not when your stress levels are higher than usual. If your enthusiasm for a new slim you is high and the timing is right, then there's no better moment than the present!

3. Set your weight-loss target. It's important to have a healthy, realistic weight-loss target in mind before starting the program. A good place to start is the BMI table on pages 16–17, not the glossy pages of a fashion or fitness magazine. Being too thin or too heavy is not good. Your health is at risk if your BMI is below 18.5 or above 24. Women, who have a lower muscle mass and smaller frame than most men, might want to target the lower end of the healthy range, say around 22; men should generally target the higher end. Remember, the BMI table is only a guide.

Those of you who have been carrying a significant amount of extra weight for a long time will have developed a stronger skeletal frame and increased muscle mass to support this extra weight, and so a BMI in the low 20s would be unrealistic. If this is the case, you will want to target the higher end of the healthy range.

The other measurement you should concern yourself with is that of your waist, which is an even better predictor of the state of your health than your weight is. Abdominal fat is more than just a weight problem. Recent research indicates that abdominal fat acts almost like a separate organ in the body, except this "organ" is a destructive one that releases harmful proteins and free fatty acids, increasing your risk of life-threatening conditions, especially heart disease.

If you are female and have a waist measurement of 35 inches or more or are male with one of over 37 inches, you are at risk of endangering your health. Women with a waist measurement of 37 inches or more and men with one over 40 inches are at serious risk of heart disease, stroke, cancer, and diabetes.

So I have your attention now! Make sure that you measure correctly: Put a tape measure around your waist just above navel level till it fits snugly, without cutting into your flesh. Do not adopt the walking-down-the-beach-sucking-in-your-stomach stance. Just stand naturally. There's no point in trying to fudge the numbers, because the only person you'll be kidding is yourself.

Now that you know your BMI and waist measurement, you can set your weight-loss target and know roughly how long it will take you to reach that goal. When you lose weight in a healthy way, you can expect to lose on average about one pound per week. I say "about" because most people do not lose weight at a fixed and steady rate. The usual pattern is to lose more at the start of the diet, when you are losing mostly water weight, followed by a series of drops and plateaus. The closer you get to your target weight, the slower your weight loss will be. If you are planning to lose up to 20 percent of your body weight—for example, if you weigh 150 pounds and want to lose 30 pounds—assume this will take you thirty weeks, one pound per week. If you have more than 20 percent to shed, the good news is that you will lose at a faster rate. This is simply because your larger body weight requires more calories just to keep operating than that of someone who is lighter. Still, be prepared for measured results—it took you a while to put on those extra pounds and it will take some time to lose them. Be patient and know that once the weight is gone, it will be gone forever as you keep it off in Phase II of the program.

Although I recommend recording your progress, please don't get obsessed with numbers on the scale. Many people find themselves losing inches before they register any weight loss. Clothes start feeling a little looser, and before you know it, you are down a dress size or getting into your old jeans. Soon you'll probably have to buy new clothes. Adherents to the G.I. Diet often tell me I should have warned them about the extra cost of refurbishing their closet!

4. Give your kitchen a green-light makeover. Take a look in your fridge—what do you see? Two jars of mayonnaise, some leftover cheddar, and a lot of sugar-laden condiments in jars? Next open the cupboards: What's the cookie and cracker situation? Now is the time to do an honest evaluation of what you tend to keep on hand. Consult the Complete G.I. Diet Food Guide (pages 290–300) and throw out anything that's in the red-light column. Be ruthless. If you have chips on hand, you will eat them. If you keep Goldfish crackers around "for the kids," you can be sure that they won't be the only ones snacking on them. Give the unopened packages and cans to a local food bank or shelter.

5. Eat before you shop. We all know what happens when you drop by the supermarket, famished, on your way home from work—before you know it, you're snacking on a bag of cookies and reaching for the biggest tray of cannelloni ever made. The worst mistake you can make is to go shopping on an empty stomach. You'll only be tempted to fill your cart with high-G.I., sugar-rich foods. If you can't swing time for a meal or snack before hitting the grocery store, pack something green-light to nibble on while you're shopping.

6. Shop green-light. For those of you who prefer a day-by-day guide to your planning, I provide a complete meal and snack plan and a grocery list for each week of the G.I. Diet Clinic in Part Two. If you'd rather not follow the plan, consult Chapter 3 to get some ideas for what to have for breakfast, lunch, dinner, and snacks during your first week on the G.I. Diet. Write a shopping list and head out to the supermarket. Your first few green-light shopping trips will require a bit more time and attention than usual as you familiarize yourself with green-light eating and meal planning. But don't worry: Before long, your new shopping and eating habits will become second nature.

Because it would be impossible to include every brand available in today's enormous supermarkets, I've listed categories of food in the G.I. Diet Food Guide rather than individual brands, except in cases where clarification is needed or where there is an especially useful product available. This means that you will have to pay some attention to food labels when comparing brands.

When reading a food label, there are six factors to consider when making the best green-light choice:

Serving Size

Is the serving size realistic, or has the manufacturer lowered it to make the calories and fat levels look better than those of the competition? When comparing brands, make sure that you are comparing the same serving size.

Calories

The product with the fewest calories is obviously the best choice.

Some products flagged as "low-fat" still have plenty of calories, so don't be fooled by the diet-friendly slogans. Calories are calories, whether they come from fat or from sugar.

Fat

Look at the amount of fat, which is often expressed as a percentage, say 2 percent (good) or 20 percent (forget it). Then check to see what sort of fat it is. You want foods that are low-fat, with minimal or no saturated and trans fats. Remember that trans fats are often called "hydrogenated oils" or "partially hydrogenated oils."

Fiber

Foods with lots of fiber have a low G.I., so when comparing brands, choose the one with higher fiber.

Sugar

Choose products that are low in sugar. Companies will sometimes quietly bump up the sugar content in foods advertised as "low-fat" to make up for any perceived loss of taste. This often happens with yogurts and cereals. Sugars are sometimes listed as corn syrup, dextrose, glucose, fructose, or sucrose; regardless of the form, it's sugar.

Sodium

Sodium (found mainly in salt) increases water retention, which doesn't help when you are trying to lose weight. It also contributes to premenstrual bloating in women and is a factor in hypertension (high blood pressure). Combine high blood pressure with excess weight and you move up to the front of the risk line for heart disease and stroke. Low-sodium products are therefore preferable.

The Recommended Dietary Allowance (RDA) for sodium is 2,500 milligrams, but this is generally regarded as too high. The National Academy of Sciences' new recommendation of 1,500 mg per day makes more sense. The average North American consumption of sodium per person per day is over 3,000 mg, so it goes without saying that most of us could stand to cut back. If you have a BMI over 30 and have any blood pressure, circulation, or heart problems, you need to be even more vigilant about seeking out low-sodium brands. Canned foods, such as soups, are often very high in sodium, as are many fast foods.

You've talked to your doctor, decided there's no better time than the present to lose weight and get healthy, set your weight-loss target, cleared your kitchen of fat-building foods, and restocked your pantry with delicious green-light choices. Now all you have to do is eat green-light meals and snacks each day, and you're well on your way to your new trim self. Following is a list of the basic green-light items you'll need in your pantry. Then, in the next section, you'll find a week-by-week guide to all the challenges and issues that will come up as you follow the G.I. Diet for the first thirteen weeks. By the end of it, you will know everything there is to know to achieve your weight-loss dreams, and you'll have lost a significant amount of weight along the way!

TO SUM UP:

The six steps to get you launched into the G.I. Diet are:

- Consult your doctor.
- Assess whether it's the right time in your life to start.
- Set your weight-loss target.
- Give your kitchen a green-light makeover.
- Eat before you shop.
- Shop green-light.

chapter five:

The G.I. Diet Clinic Pantry

BEFORE YOU GET STARTED ON THE THIRTEEN WEEKS OF THE Clinic, you'll want to take a look at the food you've got in the house. Having a well-stocked pantry makes it easy to follow a green-light diet. Here is a list of what you'll want to be sure to always have on hand at home—these items form the backbone of eating on the G.I. Diet. Use this list as a baseline for your weekly menus. Each week, you'll also find an additional grocery list for the extra ingredients needed to complete the recipes.

fruits and vegetables

apples and unsweetened applesauce
bell peppers, both red and green
mixed berries, fresh or frozen
blueberries, fresh or frozen
broccoli
carrots
celery
cucumbers
garlic
green beans
lemons
leaf lettuce
limes
mushrooms
onions, both yellow and red
oranges
mandarin oranges (no added sugar)
peaches, fresh or canned in juice or water
peas, fresh or frozen
potatoes, new or small
scallions
strawberries
plum tomatoes

dairy and deli

whole omega-3 eggs

liquid eggs or egg whites

skim milk

buttermilk (skim/1%)

hummus

nonhydrogenated, light soft margarine

low-fat sour cream

plain fat-free yogurt

fat-free fruit yogurt, with sweetener

cheese:
- Babybel Light cheese
- fat-free cottage cheese
- The Laughing Cow Light cheeses
- light feta cheese
- Parmesan cheese, grated

bakery, breakfast foods, and snacks

All-Bran Original or Bran Buds cereal

high-fiber crispbread, such as Wasa

nutrition bars, such as ZonePerfect or Balance bars

oatmeal (old-fashioned rolled oats)

100% stone-ground whole wheat bread

whole wheat pita bread

canned goods

anchovy fillets

low-fat, low-sodium chicken broth

low-fat, low-sodium vegetable broth

chickpeas

kidney beans, both red and white

lentils

diced tomatoes

plum tomatoes

stewed tomatoes

tomato paste

tomato puree

light tuna packed in water

grains and pastas

barley

bulgur

basmati rice

brown rice

small pasta, such as ditali or tubetti

whole wheat rotini or penne

herbs and spices

dried herbs:
- oregano
- thyme

fresh herbs:
- chives
- flat-leaf parsley

spices:
- ground allspice
- ground cinnamon
- chili powder
- ground cumin
- ground ginger
- ground nutmeg
- cayenne pepper
- black pepper
- red pepper flakes

salt

oils, vinegars, and condiments

fat-free mayonnaise

Dijon mustard

grainy mustard

canola oil

extra-virgin olive oil

sesame oil

vegetable cooking oil spray (canola or olive oil)

low-sodium soy sauce

steak sauce

Worcestershire sauce

tahini

cider vinegar

red wine vinegar

rice vinegar

baking ingredients

baking powder

baking soda

unsweetened cocoa powder

cornstarch

oat bran

Splenda

Sugar Twin granulated brown sugar substitute

vanilla

wheat bran

wheat germ

whole wheat flour

miscellaneous

almonds, whole and sliced

shelled, unsalted sunflower seeds

Part Two

The Thirteen-Week G.I. Diet Clinic

week 1:

Getting Started

WELCOME TO WEEK 1 OF THE G.I. DIET! BUT THIS IS MORE THAN a diet—you are starting on a journey, a new way of eating that will be how you think about food for the rest of your life. You will never have to go hungry or feel deprived. You won't have to count a single calorie or point. The extra weight will come off for as long as you eat exclusively from the long list of green-light foods in the Complete G.I. Diet Food Guide (see pages 290–300). You will feel healthy and energetic eating the nutritious green-light way. No more yo-yo dieting! It's the way to lose weight permanently.

This is the first of thirteen weeks in which I'll be working with you to change your eating habits, to overcome obstacles, and ultimately to lose excess weight. We'll discuss each week's topic, share the thoughts, worries, and victories of participants in the e-Clinic, and then close the chapter with a weekly menu and an easy-to-follow grocery list outlining all you'll need to cook green-light for the entire seven days.

The first thing I would like you to do is to fill in your current measurements and your target weight, so that you have a baseline against which to compare your progress and a place to remind yourself of your ultimate weight-loss goal. There is nothing more motivating than recording your success, so at the end of each week I will be asking you to write down your weight and waist and hip measurements. Be sure to weigh and measure yourself at the same time of day each week, since a meal or even using the bathroom can make a difference of a pound or two! I've found that an ideal time is first thing in the morning, before eating breakfast.

Current Weight: _____

Current Waist: _____

Current Hips: _____

Target Weight: _____

WHY DO YOU WANT TO LOSE WEIGHT?

Over the next thirteen weeks, I will be providing you with the knowledge, the tools, and the counsel to help make an easy transition to a new way of eating. But ultimately, for the program to work, you have to want to make it happen and you have to make the commitment to yourself. Whether it's 10 pounds or 100, it's important to look at the reasons you want to lose weight. Your answers will have a lot to do with your motivation to start and, more important, stay the course. When we started the e-Clinic, I asked the participants what their reasons were for wanting to lose weight. The following are some answers that they gave:

> *"I am a nurse who should be looking healthy and promoting a healthy lifestyle. I know that the fat that is presently around my waist is not only unattractive but unhealthy. I know that my knees would appreciate my carrying less weight."*—Marcia
>
> *"I am probably 100 pounds overweight, have high blood pressure, and am facing knee replacement surgery within the next two years. Time to get serious!"*—Karen

"I have always had a weight problem, though not to the extreme, but now as I am getting older I have noticed that my hips are sore and I don't have as much energy as I used to. Having four grandsons under five, I want to get myself in better shape to keep up with them."—Pam

"I am a 49-year-old woman who is not aging well. . . . I am always short of breath and my legs ache constantly. I was recently referred to a gastroenterologist because my blood work showed higher than normal liver enzyme counts. With a warning of the seriousness of a fatty liver, I left feeling so depressed . . . I am afraid now for my life."—Beverley

"I have been heavy all my life. . . . I remember the jokes and taunting, no proms, no dates. . . . I am an emotional eater and food has always been my comfort in times of sorrow, distress, or loneliness."—Kathy

"I know that you often read that one's appearance should not be the motivator, but it does help me to envision, this time next year, walking into a store and being able to buy a 'regular-sized' dress for the holidays."—Bernadette

"I am a blind person who has put on too much weight over the last few years. For many years I weighed 135 pounds. After the death of my parents, I found myself eating chocolate bars in the middle of the night after having numerous nightmares. The weight continued to increase and before I knew it, I was at the weight that I am now. My energy has declined and my old clothes don't fit right. I feel that just because one does not have any vision, that doesn't mean that one should look bad."—Pat

Actually, there is absolutely nothing wrong with appearance being a motivator to lose weight. In fact, it is one of the top reasons people have for wanting to slim down. Let's look at the three most common reasons people want to lose weight and see how your own reasons might be reflected.

1. I want to look better. Judging from the correspondence I have received—35,000 e-mails and counting—the day that people discover they have to dig out their "skinny" pants again is at least as rewarding as seeing the numbers fall on the scale. Most of us would rather shop for clothes that flatter and show off our bodies rather than resort to camouflage. It's a powerful motivator to walk into a room and hear a friend ask, "Have you lost weight? You look terrific." I've sold more books based on word of mouth—G.I. Diet readers being asked by friends and colleagues how they lost their weight—than through any other marketing strategy.

But wanting to look better is not just about trying to live up to unreachable, red-carpet standards of beauty or thinness: It's about feeling at ease in your body and liking what you see in the mirror. Slimming down boosts self-esteem and confidence, which in turn makes it easier to maintain new eating habits. It's amazing the difference that the loss of just a few pounds can make—not only in how you look in your clothes, but also in how you feel about yourself.

2. I want to be more energetic and to feel less lethargic. Perhaps what I hear about most frequently from readers, other than the thrill of losing pounds or going down a dress size, is the surge of energy that comes with a lighter, healthier body. Just recently, I witnessed a dramatic illustration of the kind of burden extra weight can be. My wife and I had just completed some house renovations to suit our empty-nest lifestyle, and as we were restoring some order, I asked Ruth to carry a couple of 20-pound dumbbells up a flight of stairs to my new workout room. She could get them only to the first-floor landing before she had to put them down again. "How do people who are 40 pounds overweight get around, let alone climb stairs?" she wondered. And 40 pounds of extra weight is not something you can just put down when you want to. Imagine the energy that goes into carrying those pounds! That's the energy that will be available to you again if you shed the excess weight.

Readers also tell me about the delight they experience when they find themselves able to exercise more and to enjoy activities they haven't participated in since their teens. If regaining your former energy and vitality is important to you, you'll receive constant motivation as your new, lighter body rejoices in its recently acquired freedom to run, swim, play squash, or engage in any activity you may have given up for "lack of energy."

3. I want to be healthier. Although health may not be your primary reason for losing weight, it is ultimately the most important one. Excess weight and poor diet are by far the most critical factors in increasing your chances of developing major diseases that can either undermine your quality of life or drastically shorten it. These include heart disease, stroke, cancer, diabetes, and Alzheimer's disease. Of course genes play a role in anyone's risk of these diseases, too, but people who are overweight and undernourished are putting themselves at *increased* risk for these conditions. The prospect of a long life, especially one free of pain, disability, and disease, is a powerful motivator.

I would like you to write down your own personal top three reasons for wanting to lose weight. Take a moment to be clear about your reasons, and be absolutely honest—this list is for your eyes only. Later on, come back to this page and read what you've written—it will go a long way toward keeping you motivated and helping you stick to your resolve.

My Top Three Reasons for Losing Weight

1. _____

2. _____

3. _____

FEELING A LITTLE NERVOUS?

During the first week of the e-Clinic, everyone got off to an enthusiastic start. Some participants, however, felt a little trepidation:

> *"I am afraid and nervous because nothing has worked in the past and it all seems an impossibility now. However, I am committed and will take one day at a time."*—Lynn
>
> *"I am anxious to start this new program. I look forward to the end result, which is a slimmer me. I have attempted many other diets, but I have failed."*—Pat

It's perfectly understandable if you're feeling anxious about whether you'll succeed on the G.I. Diet, particularly if you've tried and failed on diets before. But please, don't be nervous. I had failed on many diets before slimming down with green-light foods, and literally thousands of people have had great success on the G.I. Diet because this program addresses the very reasons other diets fail. The fact is that most diets really don't work. Why? I'm sure the following explanations will be familiar to you.

Why Most Diets Don't Work

1. Most diets leave you feeling hungry, weak, and deprived. You stagger through the day with a grumbling stomach, and sooner or later you cave and order a Big Mac, fries, and a shake. Feeling perpetually hungry is the primary reason that people give up on a diet.

2. The diet is too complicated and time-consuming to follow. You spend each day weighing and measuring food, calculating carbs or calories, and keeping food diaries. Perhaps this is fun initially, but then it all just becomes a burden. You're too busy to follow a diet that feels more like a math exam.

3. You feel bad. Many diets cut out essential nutrients, leaving you feeling lethargic and concerned about your health. Is it any wonder people give up?

GOALS AND REWARDS

Feeling nervous about the challenges ahead could be related to the prospect of a long journey and a considerable amount of weight to lose. If so, set a series of mini-goals for yourself. Perhaps your first mini-goal could be to lose 20 pounds, or to break the 200-pound barrier, or even to eat perfectly green-light for an entire week.

Decide what your first mini-goal will be and what you will reward yourself with once you reach that goal: A pedicure or a massage? An evening out to a movie, or that new book you've been wanting to read? Once you've reached that goal, give yourself a big pat on the back and the reward you promised yourself, and then set your next mini-goal. Setting smaller goals for yourself and reaching them will bolster your self-confidence and convince you of your ability to reach your target weight.

SUFFERING WITHDRAWAL SYMPTOMS?

During Week 1, a few participants reported feeling some unpleasant symptoms after eating green-light for a few days:

"I am finding that I am having really bad headaches since I have stopped having coffee. Up until Saturday, I would have an extra-large coffee on the way to work. I was in horrible pain today."—Tammy

"I find I am shaky and light-headed but I am not overly hungry. It is just an awful weak feeling. My hands actually shake and I feel sick. Could this be sugar withdrawal?"
—Beverley

Any major change in eating patterns requires an adjustment period, particularly when those high-sugar, high-G.I. foods are suddenly dropped from the menu. The good news is that this period of adjustment will be short because the G.I. Diet is geared to stabilize blood sugar levels, preventing those sugar highs and lows that have been a principal contributor to your weight problems.

Getting through the first week will be the hardest part. Drinking just one cup of coffee a day can cause a dependence, as can consuming caffeinated tea or soft drinks. When you suddenly put an end to your caffeine intake, you are likely to experience a headache, fatigue, a "blue" mood or irritability, and difficulty concentrating. Although these symptoms will soon pass, you may want to reduce your caffeine intake gradually, replacing half your regular coffee with decaf and then making the transition to decaf only. If you can't imagine life without your morning jolt of java, go ahead and have it, but make it just one cup a day, and use skim milk and sweetener rather than cream and sugar. By the end of the first week, you will begin to feel much better—even better than you did before you started the G.I. Diet, as Ross discovered:

> *"I stopped drinking coffee and cut out all junk food and junk snacks. Once the withdrawal symptoms passed, I started to feel more energetic. . . . I've lost 1½ inches from my waist and butt, and 1 inch from my neck. A slightly different guy (second chin shrinking) looks back at me as I shave in front of the morning mirror. . . . This program looks fantastic and realistic. For the first time ever, I feel I really can do this."*

Checking in a week later, Beverley would write:

> *"I feel much better than last week, when I wrote about the shakes and feeling weak. I actually wake up without a headache—something that has not happened in a long time."*

AT THE END OF THE WEEK

Congratulations! You've made it through the first week on the program, and you deserve a pat on the back. Below, record your weight, as well as your waist and hip measurements. Also, take the time to write about your experiences and feelings this week. Diaries help explore issues you might have to work on, ways of thinking that might be holding you back, and strategies that could work well for you.

Week 1 Weight: _____

Week 1 Waist: _____

Week 1 Hips: _____

week 1 diary

WEEK 1 OPTIONAL MEAL PLAN

	BREAKFAST	SNACK	LUNCH
MONDAY	Homey Oatmeal (p. 202) with chopped apple	Cranberry Cinnamon Bran Muffin (p. 266)	Open-faced chicken sandwich with lettuce, tomato, and onion, and Basic G.I. Salad (p. 215)
TUESDAY	Mini Breakfast Puffs (p. 206)	Fruit yogurt	G.I. Pasta Salad (p. 224)
WEDNESDAY	Homemade Muesli (p. 203) with skim milk and fruit yogurt	Cranberry Cinnamon Bran Muffin (p. 266)	½ whole wheat pita with canned light tuna, lettuce, tomato, and cucumber, and Basic G.I. Salad (p. 215)
THURSDAY	Homey Oatmeal (p. 202) with blueberries	Small apple and glass of skim milk	Quick and Easy Chicken Noodle Soup (p. 211) and Basic G.I. Salad (p. 215)
FRIDAY	All-Bran Bran Buds (or other high-fiber cereal) with skim milk, peach slices, and sliced almonds	Fruit yogurt	Mixed Bean Salad (p. 222)
SATURDAY	Western Omelet (p. 210)	½ nutrition bar	Greek Salad (p. 218)
SUNDAY	Oatmeal Buttermilk Pancakes (p. 205) with strawberries	Orange and almonds	Tuscan White Bean Soup (p. 213) and Basic G.I. Salad (p. 215)

Note: You are not required to use these weekly meal plans and shopping lists. Feel free to pick and choose and make up your own green-light meals.

SNACK	DINNER	SNACK
Laughing Cow Light cheese with crispbread	Easy-Bake Lasagna (p. 228) and Caesar Salad (p. 216)	Mixed berries tossed in lime juice with fat-free sour cream
Hummus with carrot and celery sticks	G.I. Fish Fillet (p. 237), asparagus, carrots, and new potatoes	Orange and almonds
Babybel Light cheese with crispbread	Chicken Curry (p. 247) and Raita Salad (p. 220)	Apple Pie Cookie (p. 278) and glass of skim milk
Crunchy Chickpeas (p. 271)	Vegetable Crumble (p. 230) and Tabbouleh Salad (p. 221)	½ nutrition bar
Laughing Cow Light cheese with crispbread	Fried Rice with Chicken (p. 246)	Mixed berries tossed in lime juice with fat-free sour cream
Hummus with carrot and celery sticks	Beef and Eggplant Chili (p. 257) and Basic G.I. Salad (p. 215)	Apple Pie Cookie (p. 278) and glass of skim milk
Babybel Light cheese with crispbread	Pork Medallions Dijon (p. 261), green beans, carrots, and new potatoes	Piece of Plum Crumble (p. 275)

grocery list for WEEK 1

These ingredients correspond with the recipes in this week's meal plan. Be sure that your basic pantry is well-stocked—refer to the list on pages 46–47.

produce

- ☐ asparagus
- ☐ bean sprouts
- ☐ eggplant
- ☐ kale
- ☐ leeks
- ☐ iceberg lettuce
- ☐ romaine lettuce
- ☐ fresh mint
- ☐ prune plums
- ☐ sweet potatoes
- ☐ fresh sage
- ☐ baby spinach
- ☐ fresh tarragon
- ☐ fresh thyme
- ☐ firm tofu
- ☐ zucchini

meat, poultry, and fish

- ☐ extra-lean ground beef
- ☐ pork tenderloins
- ☐ Canadian bacon
- ☐ skinless, boneless chicken breasts
- ☐ fish fillets, such as salmon or trout

dairy and deli

- ☐ low-fat cheddar cheese
- ☐ part-skim mozzarella cheese

pastas

- ☐ whole wheat lasagna
- ☐ whole wheat rotini or penne

miscellaneous

- ☐ dried cranberries
- ☐ raisins
- ☐ kalamata olives
- ☐ flax seeds
- ☐ sesame seeds
- ☐ mixed nuts
- ☐ ground cardamom
- ☐ curry powder
- ☐ low-fat tomato pasta sauce
- ☐ light tomato sauce with no added sugar

week 2:

Meal Planning

THIS WEEK I WANT TO TALK TO YOU ABOUT MEAL PLANNING and shopping for meals. One of the most important things you can do to ensure that you eat well and stick to the program is to set aside some time each week to plan your meals and snacks for the seven days ahead, as many of our e-Clinic participants discovered:

> *"I've learned there is much truth to the saying 'failing to plan is planning to fail.' In light of that, I prepared four green-light recipes last night to eat this week. Oh my goodness, they are fabulous! So I'm going into the week prepared with some really yummy and healthy foods!"*
>
> —Nancy

> *"I had a much better week. Prior planning is the key so that snacks are ready and available. A shopping plan and list has solved this problem. Also brown-bagging it is so much easier. I bought an insulated nylon lunch bag with tons of room—works great."*—Ross

> *"I plan my meals in advance for a week, due to my long commute, and adjust as necessary."*—Kathy

> *"Well, I am embarrassed about what a bad week it has been. I was not prepared for many really busy days, and I have subsequently made poor choices daily. The whole week was just one problem perpetuating another. I have told you in the past that I do feel physically better when I make better food choices, but at a time when I needed as much energy as possible, I made the worst choices. So this week I am going to try a combination of better advance planning and writing down what I eat. I am trying not to feel too discouraged, as I really want to see success with this approach, but this week has shown me that determination alone is not sufficient if you don't make other changes also."*—Bernadette

By and large, participants found that planning ahead was the key to their success on the program. If they neglected to plan, they tended to grab whatever happened to be easily available—and it usually wasn't green-light. Knowing what you are going to be eating each day and having all the ingredients at hand will not only ensure that you eat right, but also make your life simpler and put your mind at ease.

To this end, I have provided a green-light meal plan and shopping list for each week. I realize that some people enjoy cooking and trying new recipes, and others do not, so these meal plans might not be practical for everyone. It's up to you to determine what amount of planning works best for you and your lifestyle—it's different for everyone. Looking back on their thirteen weeks of the e-Clinic, Bernadette and Ross reflected on the process of adopting a meal-planning strategy that worked best for each of them. Your own plan might fall between these two extremes:

"For many weeks I struggled with the feeling that I had to start making full meals, and felt some (internal) pressure to start using recipes. But a simple approach to food preparation is working well for me and my family. . . . Fresh, homemade foods that are naturally tasty and colorful are working well for us. So we will stick to this for now."—Bernadette

"I now work out a plan for a week or so, listing the days and the meals and a possible 'menu'—nothing fancy—for example, seven breakfasts, six lunches, and six dinners to cover before the next grocery trip. Then I calculate roughly what I will need for these meals by total breakfasts, lunches, dinners, snacks—not by specific days, that's far too anal for me. This takes only a few minutes to actually do the 'math' and write the list, plus, of course, I have to actually do the shopping. Say seven breakfasts equals oatmeal for five, high-fiber cereal for two, milk, sugar substitute, so many pieces of toast, jam, fruit, etc. I calculate what I want for this meal period and time frame and buy what I need to bring the 'in home' stock up so I have no excuse to run out to the donut shop because I need breakfast but don't have time to go shopping."—Ross

Decide what will work best for you in terms of meal planning and shopping, and then make your health a priority by following through.

TURNING YOUR STANDBYS INTO GREEN-LIGHT RECIPES

You don't necessarily have to use all the recipes in this book; in fact, you can make many of your own standbys green-light by following the guidelines below.

Green-Light Ingredients

First, make sure that all the ingredients in your recipe are green-light. If there are any red- or yellow-light ingredients, either omit them or replace them with a green-light alternative.

Don't be overly rigid, though: Some red- and yellow-light foods can be used in recipes if there is a very limited quantity, such as ½ cup of wine in a dish that will serve six people, or ¼ cup of raisins in a salad for four. Full-flavored cheeses can also be used occasionally, but sparingly. For example, a tablespoon or two of grated Parmesan cheese sprinkled over a casserole will add flavor without too many calories. As long as the red- and yellow-light ingredients are used in limited quantities and not as a core ingredient, they will not have a significant impact on the overall G.I. or green-light rating of the recipe.

Fiber

The fiber content of the recipe is critical. Fiber, both soluble and insoluble, is key to the overall G.I. rating of what you eat. The more fiber, the better. If your recipe is light on fiber, consider adding boosters such as oats, bran, whole grains, or beans.

Fat

The recipe should be low in fat, with little to no saturated fat. If shortening or butter is called for, use a healthy oil or a nonhydrogenated margarine. Canola and olive oil are your best choices, but use them sparingly, because all fats are calorie-dense.

Sugar

Never add sugar or sugar-based ingredients such as corn syrup or molasses. There are some excellent sugar substitutes on the market. My favorite is Splenda, or sucralose, which was developed from a sugar base but does not have as many calories. It works well in cooking and baking. Measure it by volume (not weight) to exactly replace sugar. For example, 1 tablespoon sugar equals

1 tablespoon Splenda. Note that Splenda Brown Sugar Blend, sold for baking, is 50 percent sugar and is therefore not recommended. Brown Sugar Twin is a good alternative.

Protein

Confirm that the recipe contains sufficient protein, or that you are serving it alongside some protein to round out the meal. Protein helps slow the digestive process, which effectively lowers the G.I. of a recipe. It is also the one component that is often overlooked, particularly in recipes for salads and snacks. Useful protein boosters are low-fat dairy products; lean meats, poultry, and seafood; egg whites; beans; and soy-based foods, such as tofu and isolated soy or whey powders.

MAXIMIZING THE TIME YOU SPEND COOKING

It can be hard to find the time to cook each day, so my advice is to make big batches of green-light meals when you do have time, say on the weekends, and freeze meal-sized portions for busy nights. Having healthy meals in your freezer means you can always pull them out rather than grab a takeout menu. With a little preplanning, you won't have to rely on fast food to get you through your busy schedule! And organizing your pantry, fridge, and freezer so that they keep you going when the going gets tough will ensure the weight-loss results you want:

Week 2 Weight: _____

Week 2 Waist: _____

Week 2 Hips: _____

week 2 diary

WEEK 2 OPTIONAL MEAL PLAN

	BREAKFAST	SNACK	LUNCH
MONDAY	Homey Oatmeal (p. 202) with chopped apple	Carrot Muffin (p. 267)	Open-faced lean deli ham sandwich with lettuce, tomato, red pepper, and grainy mustard, and Basic G.I. Salad (p. 215)
TUESDAY	Mini Breakfast Puffs (p. 206)	Fruit yogurt	Waldorf Chicken and Rice Salad (p. 226)
WEDNESDAY	Homemade Muesli (p. 203) with skim milk and fruit yogurt	Carrot Muffin (p. 267)	Cottage cheese with apple and grapes, and Basic G.I. Salad (p. 215)
THURSDAY	Homey Oatmeal (p. 202) with blueberries	Small apple and glass of skim milk	Minestrone (p. 212) and Basic G.I. Salad (p. 215)
FRIDAY	All-Bran Bran Buds (or other high-fiber cereal) with skim milk, peach slices, and sliced almonds	Fruit yogurt	½ whole wheat pita with deli turkey, lettuce, tomato, and cucumber, and Basic G.I. Salad (p. 215)
SATURDAY	Italian Omelet (p. 208)	½ nutrition bar	Crab Salad in Tomato Shells (p. 225)
SUNDAY	Cinnamon French Toast (p. 204) with Canadian bacon	Orange and almonds	Ham and Lentil Soup (p. 214) and Basic G.I. Salad (page 215)

Note: You are not required to use these weekly meal plans and shopping lists. Feel free to pick and choose and make up your own green-light meals.

SNACK	DINNER	SNACK
Laughing Cow Light cheese with crispbread	Fettuccine Primavera (p. 227) and Caesar Salad (p. 216)	Mixed berries tossed in lime juice with fat-free sour cream
Hummus with carrot and celery sticks	Ginger-Wasabi Halibut (p. 240), Cold Noodle Salad with Cucumber and Sesame (p. 223), snow peas and carrots	Orange and almonds
Babybel Light cheese with crispbread	Chicken Tarragon with Mushrooms (p. 245), broccoli, and basmati rice	Pecan Brownie (p. 280) and glass of skim milk
Crunchy Chickpeas (p. 271)	Meat Loaf (p. 259), green beans, carrots, and new potatoes	½ nutrition bar
Laughing Cow Light cheese with crispbread	Bean and Onion Pizza (p. 234)	Mixed berries tossed in lime juice with fat-free sour cream
Hummus with carrot and celery sticks	Grilled Tuna with Chimichurri Sauce (p. 241), asparagus, and new potatoes	Pecan Brownie (p. 280) and glass of skim milk
Babybel Light cheese with crispbread	Orange Chicken with Almonds (p. 250), green beans, and basmati rice	Slice of Apple Raspberry Coffee Cake (p. 272)

grocery list for WEEK 2

These ingredients correspond with the recipes in this week's meal plan. Be sure that your basic pantry is well-stocked—refer to the list on pages 46–47.

produce

- ☐ asparagus
- ☐ fresh basil
- ☐ fresh cilantro
- ☐ fresh ginger
- ☐ grapes
- ☐ raspberries
- ☐ snow peas
- ☐ romaine lettuce
- ☐ baby spinach
- ☐ firm tofu
- ☐ large beefsteak tomatoes
- ☐ yellow summer squash

meat, poultry, and fish

- ☐ extra-lean ground beef
- ☐ Canadian bacon
- ☐ skinless, boneless chicken breasts
- ☐ canned crab
- ☐ halibut fillets
- ☐ tuna steaks, ½ inch thick

dairy and deli

- ☐ part-skim mozzarella cheese
- ☐ low-fat, low-sugar buttermilk salad dressing
- ☐ lean deli ham
- ☐ lean deli turkey

pastas

- ☐ whole wheat capellini or spaghettini
- ☐ whole wheat fettuccine or linguine

miscellaneous

- ☐ active dry yeast
- ☐ dried tarragon
- ☐ sun-dried tomatoes
- ☐ raisins
- ☐ flax seeds
- ☐ sesame seeds
- ☐ pecans
- ☐ walnuts
- ☐ wasabi powder
- ☐ mirin or sweet sherry
- ☐ low-fat tomato pasta sauce
- ☐ tomato juice
- ☐ vegetable cocktail juice

week 3:

Behavior Change

THIS WEEK WAS CLEARLY A PERIOD OF ADJUSTMENT AS E-CLINIC participants became more aware of their eating habits and came to terms with the day-to-day realities of changing them:

> *"Finishing things the kids have left on their plates has become such an established habit for me that there were times I was shocked to see myself on 'autopilot' just doing this, even when I wasn't hungry."*—Bernadette
>
> *"I had a good week but found that eating breakfast is the hardest thing for me to do. I am not really hungry, so I am choking down high-fiber cereal at my desk at seven in the morning. The weekend was better because I had time to make oatmeal, and you are right, it stays with you a lot longer than anything else."*—Beverley
>
> *"I found out that, for me, nuts can't be a snack. It is too easy to take a handful of cashews and almonds rather than the suggested amount, or to pop one or two extra as I count out the correct amount."*—Kathy

"I think where I went wrong this week was not eating enough small snacks. As a matter of fact, I often skipped the snacks, thinking that would help me in the long run . . . and more weight would be lost. Boy, I sure got fooled."—Pat

"Weekends are the hardest for me, as I don't have the structure of my workday with break time and lunch, so I may have to resort to a timer or alarm to remind me to eat. I usually end up not eating much at all throughout the day, then realizing I didn't eat very much and then having a slightly larger than normal dinner. I simply forget to eat as I don't feel hungry—I get busy with doing things around the house or out and about and it doesn't occur to me to eat something."—Kimberley

Kimberley has an excellent idea there! If you are having trouble remembering to eat all your snacks and meals, why don't you buy a cheap watch with an alarm that you can set to remind yourself to eat. When you skip snacks or meals, all you do is end up eating more—not less—by day's end.

BREAKING BAD HABITS

Let's face it: Change isn't always easy, and old habits can be hard to break. But to lose a significant amount of weight permanently, it is absolutely necessary to ditch those habits that led to the weight gain in the first place. Simply modifying your existing way of eating won't do it; you have to rethink your priorities and be willing to make fundamental changes in the way you approach food and eating. Making the commitment to commit is half the battle; making the necessary life changes is the rest.

To ease the transition, bad habits will need to be replaced with good habits that you can easily handle. The following is a list of the top ten bad habits that prevent weight loss and what can be done to change them.

1. Skipping Breakfast It is estimated that one quarter of North Americans skip breakfast, and the numbers are even worse for teenagers—a study of U.S. teens showed that only 32 percent were eating breakfast regularly! Breakfast is the most important meal of the day: By the time people rise in the morning, most haven't eaten for ten to twelve hours, and their blood sugar levels are low. As a result skipping breakfast will most certainly cause you to snack throughout the day in an effort to boost your blood sugar, or energy, level. And chances are good that you will reach for high-calorie, high-fat foods such as doughnuts, muffins, or cookies to give you that quick sugar fix your body feels it needs. But we are all well aware by now that the blood sugar high caused by these red-light foods will soon be followed by a sugar crash as your insulin kicks in, and you'll be looking for your next sugar fix.

It's tremendously important that you never skip breakfast. Research consistently shows that people who eat breakfast actually eat fewer calories per day and lose weight more successfully than those who do not. Always start your day with a substantial breakfast.

2. Not Taking Time to Eat Properly Saying "I don't have time to eat properly" creates a spawning ground for bad habits. People who don't take the time to eat properly tend to grab a coffee and pastry on their way to work, eat a store-bought muffin midmorning to boost flagging energy levels, have a slice or two of pizza with Coke for lunch, snack on chocolate and cookies in the afternoon to help keep their eyes open, pick up some high-fat take-out food on the way home for dinner, and finally collapse in front of the TV for the evening with beer and a bowl of pretzels.

It's easy to slip into this harmful cycle of fattening convenience foods and short-term energy fixes, but you'll pay for the convenience with a growing girth, flagging energy, and poor health. And really, the amount of incremental time required to prepare your own healthy meals and snacks is quite modest. Fifteen minutes in the morning is all it takes to prepare and eat a healthy breakfast—often the length of time it takes to wait in line at the coffee shop. If you can't manage to squeeze in a nutritious breakfast before rushing off to work, then take along a box of green-light cereal, a carton of skim milk, and a piece of fruit. Another piece of fruit and a carton of skim milk for later in the day takes no time to prepare and makes a filling, nutritious snack. And there are always places where you can get a green-light sandwich or salad so you don't resort to pizza. Eating healthfully throughout the day will ensure that, when you arrive at home, you have the energy to prepare a quick green-light dinner in the time it would have taken to drive to the take-out place and wait for your order. A little extra time and thought is all that's required to break out of the "I don't have time . . ." habits—for good.

3. Grazing The world's best grazers are teenagers. They simply cannot avoid opening the fridge every time they pass it. Their rapid growth and (hopefully) high activity levels require a constant high-calorie intake. Unfortunately, grazing is a habit that many people continue into their adult lives, with disastrous results for their waistlines and health. A few nuts here, a couple of cookies there, a tablespoon or two of peanut butter, and a few glasses of juice all look pretty harmless in themselves, but taken together they can easily total several hundred extra calories a day! And those can add up to over 20 pounds of additional weight in a year.

On the G.I. Diet, you should be eating three meals plus three to four snacks a day, which means you are eating something approximately every two hours during your waking hours. This will reduce your temptation to graze. One reader wrote that she couldn't believe how she could be losing weight when she always seemed to be eating. She called it "green-light grazing"!

4. Unconscious Eating How often have we begun to nibble on a bowl of chips or nuts or a box of cookies while watching TV, reading a book, or talking on the phone and then suddenly realized that we'd eaten the whole lot? Too often, I would guess. Eating should never be a peripheral activity—it should always be the focus. Eat your meals at the table and set aside distractions such as the TV, computer, video game, or telephone while you have your snacks. This will help you to always eat consciously and to be aware of exactly how much you are eating—and when to stop.

5. Eating Too Quickly The famous Horace Fletcher is said to have asserted at the turn of the eighteenth century that food should always be chewed thirty-two times before swallowing. Though this seems rather excessive, there is an important truth here. Many of us tend to eat far too quickly. It takes twenty to thirty minutes for the stomach to let the brain know it is full. If you eat too quickly, you'll continue to eat past the point at which you've had enough. The solution, then, is to eat slowly to allow your brain to catch up with your stomach. That's probably another reason that France has a substantially lower rate of obesity (less than half that of the U.S.): The French take far longer to eat their meals. There, mealtimes are for family and friends, and for enjoying the pleasure of food—not simply a means to tackle hunger. To ensure you are not eating more than your appetite requires, slow down and really enjoy what you are eating. Put your fork down between mouthfuls. Savor the flavors and textures.

6. Not Drinking Enough Did you know that by the time you feel thirsty you are already dehydrated? Your body's need for water is second only to its need for oxygen. Up to 70 percent of the body is water, and we should be drinking about eight glasses a day to replenish our supply. Yet many of us don't take the time to drink enough, and we go through our days in a mild state of dehydration. Being dehydrated makes us feel tired and hungry, which makes us reach for food when really we should be reaching for a glass of water. Our bodies aren't hungry, they're thirsty. So always carry a water bottle with you and make sure you are drinking the recommended amount. Being properly hydrated will go a long way toward helping you control your appetite and lose weight. If you're not much of a water drinker, try sipping on iced herbal tea (unsweetened, or with a sweetener such as Splenda), calorie-free flavored sparkling water, or even diet caffeine-free soda.

7. Over-Rewarding for Exercise Another common bad habit is to reward yourself with food for doing some exercise—often resulting in the consumption of more calories than you've just burned. Even a rewarding latte after your workout can wipe out all that hard work. Though exercise is essential for long-term health and weight maintenance, it is actually a poor tool for *losing* weight—and its benefits are quickly offset by red- or yellow-light snacking. To give you an idea of how much you would have to exercise to lose just one pound of fat, you would have to walk briskly for *forty-two* miles if you weighed 160 pounds or *fifty-three miles* if you weighed 130 pounds. That is a huge amount of effort and way beyond the capability or time availability of most people. Walking around the block or washing the car consumes only a handful of calories. So if you are using exercise as permission to cut a little slack in your diet, remember that that cookie reward will add more calories than you expended on your activity.

By all means exercise to improve your health, but don't think it will contribute a whole lot to your weight loss. I frequently tell people that losing weight is 90 percent diet and 10 percent exercise, particularly in the early stages. (For more on exercise, see Week 12.)

8. Cleaning Your Plate Many of us were taught from the time we were small to finish what's on our plates before leaving the table. This becomes a deeply embedded habit that, unfortunately, does not help lose or maintain weight in later life. And not only do we finish our own, but we tend to also finish the leftovers on our children's plates or that last lonely slice in the pie dish after dinner. I confess that I do! But this habit causes us to eat more than we need to satisfy our hunger and is therefore dreadful for weight control. Get into the habit of letting your stomach and brain decide when you are full, not the quantity of food on your plate. Leftovers can always be stored in the fridge rather than around your waist and hips.

If you find yourself struggling with this, a quick solution can be to simply use smaller plates! Our brains react much more favorably to a small plate that's full of food than to a large plate that's sparsely filled.

9. Shopping on an Empty Stomach Human nature can often be perverse, encouraging us to do the right thing but at the wrong time. When you are full and satisfied, food shopping is rarely top of mind. But when you are hungry, it suddenly seems like a very good idea indeed. Unfortunately, it isn't: You'll end up with a shopping cart that has been filled by your stomach rather than by your head. Those red-light foods will seem far more tempting than usual, and you will probably make some poor choices as a result.

Avoid temptation by shopping after a meal, or at least take a portable green-light snack, such as a muffin or nutrition bar, with you. Another smart idea is to take along a detailed shopping list and stick to it! You'll make far wiser choices this way.

10. Eating High-Sugar, High-Fat Treats Food is a big part of holidays and celebrations—just think of Thanksgiving, a wedding, a bar mitzvah, or Christmas and you'll probably picture the special foods that go along with them. Where would the candy industry be without Valentine's Day, Halloween, or Easter? Food is often linked with positive experiences, which is one reason we often think of certain foods as "treats." And it's not just holidays: Whether it's Granny doling out candies to a child who has been good or a neighbor with a freshly baked pie for raking up her leaves, we are accustomed to using food treats to reward the people in our lives as well as ourselves.

Unfortunately, these so-called treats tend to be high in calories, sugar, and fat, and certainly are not our friends. They are, in fact, a major contributor to the obesity crisis and to weight-related diseases such as diabetes and heart disease. We really should start to view these foods as penalties rather than rewards.

If you must indulge your sweet tooth, choose treats that are lower in calories and fat. If candy is your thing, there is a plethora of low- and no-sugar brands available. Fresh fruit and low-fat, no-sugar-added yogurt and ice cream are even better treats. And there are many delicious green-light dessert and snack recipes in all my G.I. Diet books, including this one. Treats are a wonderful part of our lives—just make sure they are the right sort of treats.

Keep in mind that while changing bad habits will take some effort and will be challenging at times, it's well worth your while to persevere with these beneficial new behaviors. Before you know it, they'll be second nature, as firmly entrenched as the old ones used to be, but these will help you slim down to a brand-new you. To end this week on a positive note, here are some observations from e-Clinic participants as they completed Week 3 of the program:

"The weight is coming off so easily, I am really excited."
—Tammy

"I feel more energetic for sure, and loose pants are still in fashion so I won't need new pants just yet."—Ross

Week 3 Weight: _____

Week 3 Waist: _____

Week 3 Hips: _____

week 3 diary

WEEK 3 OPTIONAL MEAL PLAN

	BREAKFAST	SNACK	LUNCH
MONDAY	Homey Oatmeal (p. 202) with chopped apple	Apple Bran Muffin (p. 264)	Open-faced chicken sandwich with lettuce, tomato, and onion, and Basic G.I. Salad (p. 215)
TUESDAY	Mini Breakfast Puffs (p. 206)	Fruit yogurt	G.I. Pasta Salad (p. 224)
WEDNESDAY	Homemade Muesli (p. 203) with skim milk and fruit yogurt	Apple Bran Muffin (p. 264)	½ whole wheat pita with canned light tuna, lettuce, tomato, and cucumber, and Basic G.I. Salad (p. 215)
THURSDAY	Homey Oatmeal (p. 202) with blueberries	Small apple and glass of skim milk	Quick and Easy Chicken Noodle Soup (p. 211) and Basic G.I. Salad (p. 215)
FRIDAY	All-Bran Bran Buds (or other high-fiber cereal) with skim milk, peach slices, and sliced almonds	Fruit yogurt	Mixed Bean Salad (p. 222)
SATURDAY	Vegetarian Omelet (p. 209)	½ nutrition bar	Greek Salad (p. 218)
SUNDAY	Oatmeal Buttermilk Pancakes (p. 205) with strawberries	Orange and almonds	Tuscan White Bean Soup (p. 213) and Basic G.I. Salad (p. 215)

Note: You are not required to use these weekly meal plans and shopping lists. Feel free to pick and choose and make up your own green-light meals.

SNACK	DINNER	SNACK
Laughing Cow Light cheese with crispbread	Rigatoni with Mini Meatballs (p. 254) and Caesar Salad (p. 216)	Mixed berries tossed in lime juice with fat-free sour cream
Hummus with carrot and celery sticks	Citrus-Poached Haddock (p. 239), green beans, and new potatoes	Orange and almonds
Babybel Light cheese with crispbread	Chicken Jambalaya (p. 256) and broccoli	Creamy Lemon Square (p. 279) and glass of skim milk
Crunchy Chickpeas (p. 271)	Barley Risotto with Leeks, Lemon, and Peas (p. 236) and Tabbouleh Salad (p. 221)	½ nutrition bar
Laughing Cow Light cheese with crispbread	Thai Red Curry Shrimp Pasta (p. 244)	Mixed berries tossed in lime juice with fat-free sour cream
Hummus with carrot and celery sticks	Zesty Barbecued Chicken (p. 252), Tangy Red and Green Coleslaw (p. 219), and new potatoes	Creamy Lemon Square (p. 279) and glass of skim milk
Babybel Light cheese with crispbread	Pork Tenderloin with Apple Compote (p. 260), brussels sprouts, carrots, and new potatoes	Piece of Berry Crumble (p. 274)

grocery list for WEEK 3

These ingredients correspond with the recipes in this week's meal plan. Be sure that your basic pantry is well-stocked—refer to the list on pages 46–47.

produce

- ☐ brussels sprouts
- ☐ cabbage, both green and red
- ☐ fresh cilantro
- ☐ eggplant
- ☐ kale
- ☐ leeks
- ☐ iceberg lettuce
- ☐ romaine lettuce
- ☐ fresh mint
- ☐ fresh rosemary
- ☐ fresh sage
- ☐ zucchini

meat, poultry, and fish

- ☐ pork tenderloin
- ☐ skinless, boneless chicken breasts
- ☐ lean ground chicken or turkey
- ☐ haddock fillets
- ☐ large raw shrimp

dairy and deli

- ☐ low-fat cheddar cheese

pastas

- ☐ whole wheat macaroni or small shells
- ☐ whole wheat rigatoni
- ☐ whole wheat rotini or penne
- ☐ whole wheat spaghettini or linguine

miscellaneous

- ☐ ground almonds
- ☐ ground cloves
- ☐ pecans
- ☐ flax seeds
- ☐ celery seeds
- ☐ dried currants
- ☐ kalamata olives
- ☐ bay leaves
- ☐ dried sage
- ☐ Thai red curry paste
- ☐ light tomato sauce with no added sugar
- ☐ frozen apple juice concentrate
- ☐ unsweetened apple juice
- ☐ unsweetened orange juice

week 4:

Falling Off the Wagon

FALLING OFF THE WAGON IS BOUND TO HAPPEN SOONER OR later. And while I don't encourage it, as long as it's the exception and not the rule, it's acceptable. This diet isn't meant to be a straitjacket, after all. If you do your best to eat the green-light way 90 percent of the time, you'll still lose weight. The odd lapse, at worst, will delay you by a week or two from reaching your target weight. So don't be so hard on yourself; just be sure to get right back on the plan with the next meal.

Some people make the mistake of feeling so bad about slipping up that they just give up. But you should anticipate that you *will* fall off the wagon from time to time. The best way to handle it is to learn why it happened and decide how you will handle the situation the next time. Rather than dwell on the negative, think about the positive, as Ross did:

> *"There was a family dinner party with Chinese food where I strayed, but remarkably I only had one medium plate and not the usual two heaping plates of food I would have had in the past. Also, I felt no hunger pains when I didn't have the extra food this time—a definite change."*

Here's how the other e-Clinic participants dealt with their occasional slip-ups:

"Two lessons from this week: (1) Keep green-light food handy and (2) the weight goes back on a whole lot easier than it comes off."—Karen

"This past week has been really good, although I had a couple of functions where I couldn't follow the diet to the tee (I had a couple of alcoholic drinks and chicken strips with fries and ketchup). The next day, it was back to the diet. I felt extremely guilty, but my friends and family told me that it's okay to indulge once in a while, as long as I keep with my diet the rest of the time, which I do."—Tammy

"Last night I made a batch of cookies for a coworker's birthday and was ridiculously hard on myself for eating one cookie. When I changed my perspective, however, I realized that just a few weeks ago I would've eaten about a dozen of those cookies and then beat myself up for having done so. Plus, eating that cookie made me think about trade-offs: Would I rather eat the cookie or go off my plan in some other way, or would I prefer to use a bit of 'wiggle room' to enjoy a glass of wine with dinner one night? There again, I can see that my perspective is changing, and that is of utmost importance for me to succeed, in my opinion."—Nancy

"I have come to learn over years of dieting that if you slip up and make a bad choice, you need to get back on track ASAP, as one mistake can quietly transform into a week of mistakes. I think that process of reestablishing your focus must be critical in successful weight loss."—Bernadette

Several participants said that the hardest part of the day was the evening, when they had the most difficulty steering clear of temptation. Some, like Ross, used green-light snacks to help them:

> *"I have my hardest time after work during prime snacking time, which was a major downfall period previously. I have put two of my snack times in here. I have managed to eat just green-light snacks, but some nights I still have cravings for the bad stuff. I feel like I imagine an alcoholic does on many nights."*

Although most people find that their cravings do diminish after a few weeks on the G.I. Diet, there will still be times when a craving will surface because of the leveling effects that green-light eating has on one's blood sugar levels. Here's how to handle the situation:

1. Try to distract yourself with an activity. Call a friend, fold a basket of laundry, take out the garbage, or just go for a walk. Sometimes a craving will pass.

2. If you're still having the craving, pinpoint the flavor you want and find a green-light food that has it. For example, if it's something sweet, have strawberries or applesauce; if you want something sweet and creamy, try low-fat yogurt or ice cream with no added sugar; if you want something salty, have a couple of olives or a dill pickle, or some hummus with veggies; if it's chocolate you want, try half of a chocolate-flavored nutrition bar or a mug of light instant hot chocolate. There are many green-light versions of the foods we normally reach for when a craving strikes.

3. Sometimes nothing but a piece of chocolate or a spoonful of peanut butter will do. If this is the case, have a small portion and really enjoy it. Eat it *slowly* and savor the experience. Chalk it up to that 10 percent leeway you're allowed on the G.I. Diet. Just make sure you're staying green-light 90 percent of the time.

The good news is that as you continue with your green-light eating, you'll find yourself getting better and better at resisting those bad old foods. Have a look at what e-Clinic participants had to say:

"I'm finding the cravings diminishing since working on this diet, and driving by the fast-food places is less tempting as well. I'm encouraged that I can take more control over my eating, which is a relief to my wife!"—J. V.

"Except for the one week I was away, plus the wedding, the weight is coming off. I keep expecting to get on the scale and see it's all a mistake. How is it possible to lose five pounds in one week? This has never happened in the past! Don't get me wrong, I'm pleased, but it seems like it's too good to be true."—Lynn

"It doesn't seem like I'm really on a diet (or doing a 'lifestyle change') in general. There are still the occasional times when I have a craving for a Hershey chocolate bar. During times like those, there is a yellow-light quick fix. That's when I'll take a small piece of my wife's organic 70 percent cocoa chocolate bar. It is just enough to take away the craving (the bitterness helps), and I stay on the green-light track the rest of the time."—J

Week 4 Weight: _____

Week 4 Waist: _____

Week 4 Hips: _____

week 4 diary

WEEK 4 OPTIONAL MEAL PLAN

	BREAKFAST	SNACK	LUNCH
MONDAY	Homey Oatmeal (p. 202) with chopped apple	Whole Wheat Fruit Scone (p. 269)	Open-faced lean deli ham sandwich with lettuce, tomato, red pepper, and grainy mustard, and Basic G.I. Salad (p. 215)
TUESDAY	Mini Breakfast Puffs (p. 206)	Fruit yogurt	Waldorf Chicken and Rice Salad (p. 226)
WEDNESDAY	Homemade Muesli (p. 203) with skim milk and fruit yogurt	Whole Wheat Fruit Scone (p. 269)	Cottage cheese with apple and grapes, and Basic G.I. Salad (p. 215)
THURSDAY	Homey Oatmeal (p. 202) with blueberries	Small apple and glass of skim milk	Minestrone (p. 212) and Basic G.I. Salad (p. 215)
FRIDAY	All-Bran Bran Buds (or other high-fiber cereal) with skim milk, peach slices, and sliced almonds	Fruit yogurt	½ whole wheat pita with deli turkey, lettuce, tomato, and cucumber, and Basic G.I. Salad (p. 215)
SATURDAY	Canadian Bacon Omelet (p. 207)	½ nutrition bar	Crab Salad in Tomato Shells (p. 225)
SUNDAY	Cinnamon French Toast (p. 204) with Canadian bacon	Orange and almonds	Ham and Lentil Soup (p. 214) and Basic G.I. Salad (p. 215)

Note: You are not required to use these weekly meal plans and shopping lists. Feel free to pick and choose and make up your own green-light meals.

SNACK	DINNER	SNACK
Laughing Cow Light cheese with crispbread	Salmon Pasta (p. 238)	Mixed berries tossed in lime juice with fat-free sour cream
Hummus with carrot and celery sticks	Pan-Seared Whitefish with Mandarin Salsa (p. 242), broccoli, and basmati rice	Orange and almonds
Babybel Light cheese with crispbread	Chicken Schnitzel (p. 248), green beans, carrots, and new potatoes	Slice of Strawberry Tea Bread (p. 270) and glass of skim milk
Crunchy Chickpeas (p. 271)	Mushroom Gravy Pork Chops (p. 263), asparagus, and basmati rice	½ nutrition bar
Laughing Cow Light cheese with crispbread	Horseradish Burgers (p. 258) and Tabbouleh Salad (p. 221)	Mixed berries tossed in lime juice with fat-free sour cream
Hummus with carrot and celery sticks	Vegetarian Moussaka (p. 232) and basmati rice	Slice of Strawberry Tea Bread (p. 270) and glass of skim milk
Babybel Light cheese with crispbread	Spicy Roast Chicken with Tomatoes and Tarragon (p. 249), green beans, and basmati rice	Slice of One-Bowl Chocolate Cake (p. 276)

grocery list for WEEK 4

These ingredients correspond with the recipes in this week's meal plan. Be sure that your basic pantry is well-stocked—refer to the list on pages 46–47.

produce

- ☐ alfalfa sprouts (optional)
- ☐ asparagus
- ☐ fresh basil
- ☐ fresh cilantro
- ☐ grapes
- ☐ fresh mint
- ☐ baby spinach
- ☐ fresh tarragon
- ☐ large beefsteak tomatoes
- ☐ cherry or grape tomatoes

meat, poultry, and fish

- ☐ extra-lean ground beef
- ☐ boneless pork loin chops
- ☐ Canadian bacon
- ☐ skinless, boneless chicken breasts
- ☐ whitefish fillets
- ☐ canned crab
- ☐ salmon fillet

dairy and deli

- ☐ low-fat, low-sugar buttermilk salad dressing
- ☐ light herb and garlic cream cheese
- ☐ lean deli ham
- ☐ lean deli turkey

pastas

- ☐ whole wheat macaroni or small shells

miscellaneous

- ☐ dried apricots
- ☐ dried basil
- ☐ Italian herb seasoning
- ☐ prepared horseradish
- ☐ sun-dried tomatoes
- ☐ pecans
- ☐ walnuts
- ☐ unsweetened apple juice
- ☐ unsweetened orange juice
- ☐ whole wheat bread crumbs
- ☐ whole wheat hamburger buns

week 5:

Eating Out

IT'S HIGH TIME WE DEALT WITH THE TRICKY ISSUE OF EATING out. I say tricky because, unlike when you eat at home, in restaurants you have little control over what goes into the meals and how they are prepared. Nevertheless, there are ways in which you can minimize any potential damage.

Over the past twenty years or so, there has been a dramatic increase in serving sizes—a phenomenon termed "portion distortion." Let me give you some examples from a survey of restaurant portions prepared by the National Heart, Lung, and Blood Institute:

	20 YEARS AGO		TODAY	
Snacks	**Size**	**Calories**	**Size**	**Calories**
Bagel	3 inches	140	6 inches	350
French fries	2.4 ounces	210	7 ounces	610
Muffin	1.5 ounces	210	5 ounces	500
Cookie	1.5 inches	55	4 inches	275
Meals				
Spaghetti & meatballs		500		1,025
Turkey sandwich		320		820
Chicken Caesar salad		390		700
Chicken stir-fry		435		865

As you can see, the size and corresponding calories of food have doubled or even tripled over a relatively short period. And we have come to accept these new super-sized portions as standard. A study done with Canadian college students on their consumption of their favorite food, macaroni and cheese, shows that the more that was put in front of them, the more they ate. Yet they reported that they felt no fuller on the larger portions than on the smaller ones. Moral: If it's not on your plate, you won't miss it.

Challenges: Eating Out While Traveling

It is essential to plan ahead when traveling, because lack of access to kitchens or grocery stores can leave you entirely at the mercy of a restaurant menu. When I am on the road during media tours, I frequently find myself in situations where there is no green-light food in sight. Just in case, I always carry emergency green-light reserves with me, such as nuts, nutrition bars (usually Balance Bars), homemade green-light muffins, and fruit.

Breakfast tends to be the biggest challenge of the day because I habitually eat it wherever I'm staying, as most people do. (For lunch and dinner, there is usually a wider choice of venue and menu.) Fortunately, oatmeal appears to be increasingly available in hotels. Failing that, look for high-fiber cereals, yogurt, and fruit. Skim milk is normally available on request. As a last resort, I always carry a couple of pouches of plain instant oatmeal with me, which require only the addition of hot water. Though this option is not as good as the oatmeal you make from scratch, it's certainly better than sugary breakfast cereal!

If you can find a solution to deal with snacks and breakfast, then staying green-light while traveling is definitely doable. For lunch and dinner, keep an eye on my tips for dining out, which follow.

TOP TEN TIPS FOR DINING OUT

Although supersize portions and three-course meal deals may look like a terrific value, just think what they have cost us in terms of extra pounds and poorer health. Difficult though it may be to refrain from eating everything that has been placed in front of you—I certainly suffer from this—moderation and common sense are your waistline's best friends. Don't feel guilty about leaving food on your plate!

In addition to this fundamental recommendation, here are my top ten tips for dining out with family and friends the green-light way:

1. Just before you go out, have a small bowl of high-fiber, green-light cold cereal (such as All-Bran) with skim milk and sweetener. I often add a couple of spoonfuls of no-fat/no-sugar fruit yogurt. This will take the edge off your appetite and get some fiber into your digestive system, which will help reduce the G.I. of your upcoming meal.

2. Once seated in the restaurant, drink a glass of water. It will help you feel fuller.

3. Once the basket of rolls or bread—which you will ignore—has been passed around the table, ask the server to remove it. The longer it sits there, the more tempted you will be to dig in.

4. Order a soup or salad first and tell the server you would like it as soon as possible. This will keep you from sitting there hungry while others are filling up on the bread. For soups, go for vegetable- or bean-based, the chunkier the better. Avoid anything that is cream-based, and don't be nervous about asking whether an unfamiliar soup contains cream. For salads, the golden rule is to keep the dressing on the side. Then you can use a fraction of what the restaurant would normally pour over the greens. Avoid Caesar salads, which come pre-dressed and often pack as many calories as a burger.

5. Since you probably won't get boiled new potatoes and can't be sure of what type of rice is being served, ask for double vegetables instead of a starchy side dish. I have yet to find a restaurant that won't oblige.

6. Stick with low-fat cuts of meat or poultry. If necessary, remove the skin before eating. Duck is usually too high in fat to count as green-light. Fish and shellfish are excellent choices but shouldn't be breaded or battered. Tempura is more fat and flour than filling. Remember that servings tend to be generous in restaurants, so eat only 4 to 6 ounces (the size of a pack of cards) and leave the rest.

7. As with salads, ask for any sauces for your meat to be served on the side.

8. Remember to eat slowly to allow your brain the time it needs to realize you're full. Put your fork down between mouthfuls and savor your meal.

9. For dessert, fresh fruit and berries—without the ice cream—are your best choice. Most other desserts are a dietary disaster. If you don't have the choice of fruit, my advice is to avoid dessert entirely. If a birthday cake is being passed around, share your piece with someone. A couple of forkfuls or so along with your coffee should get you off the hook, with minimal dietary damage!

10. Order only decaffeinated coffee. Skim milk decaf cappuccino is my family's favorite after-dinner choice.

FAST FOOD

Not so long ago, the idea of getting a green-light lunch at a fast-food outlet was simply laughable. Now, however, partly due to the threat of legal action and a stagnant market share, the major fast-food chains are finally offering some healthy options. Subway has been pioneering the move toward healthy choices for some time, and its initiative has been reflected in its successful growth.

Although things are changing, fast food is still a minefield. Hamburgers are soaked in saturated fat, as are deep-fried chicken and fish. The trimmings—fries, ketchup, shakes, and regular soft drinks—are loaded with fat and sugar.

I recommend avoiding pizza restaurants like the plague, since pizza generally has high-G.I. crust and lots of saturated fat in the cheese toppings. However, it's increasingly common to see salads on the menu, so it might be worth calling the restaurant ahead of time to find out if there are some green-light options available besides the high-G.I. pizza.

Below I've listed other good choices in fast food. An asterisk indicates items that are excessively high in sodium—the fast-food industry frequently boosts salt content when lowering fat to make up for any perceived loss of flavor—which can be hazardous to your health.

Note: This information was correct at time of publication. However, because fast-food restaurants make frequent menu changes, you may wish to check their menus or websites from time to time to see if they have expanded their green-light offerings.

Ground Rules

1. Always eat burgers and sandwiches open-faced, throwing away the top half of the bun.

2. Always ask for low-fat dressings, and even then use only half the packet.

SUBWAY

Subway has been the pacesetter in the fast-food industry with its broad range of low-fat foods. As a mark of its success, the chain now has more retail outlets than McDonald's has.

Sandwiches (Subs): 6 inches/6g of fat

All sandwiches should include bread, lettuce, tomatoes, onions, green peppers, pickles, and olives. Best choice of roll is Wheat or Honey Oat.

- Ham*
- Roast Beef*
- Turkey Breast*
- Chicken Breast*
- Veggie Delite

If high blood pressure is a concern, use only fat-free honey mustard or sweet onion sauces, and replace pickles and olives with cucumbers and onions.

Wrap

- Veggie Delite

Salads: 6g of fat or less

- All salads except Ham, Subway Club, and Turkey Breast and Ham

Dressing

- Fat-free Italian

MCDONALD'S

Sandwiches

- Premium Grilled Chicken Classic* (Replace the mayo with half a packet of BBQ sauce.)

*high salt content

Salads

- Asian Salad with Grilled Chicken
- Bacon Ranch Salad with Grilled Chicken
- Caesar Salad with Grilled Chicken
- Fruit and Walnut Salad
- Premium Southwest Salad with Grilled Chicken

Dressings

- Newman's Own Low-Fat Balsamic Vinaigrette*
- Newman's Own Low-Fat Family Recipe Italian*
- Newman's Own Low-Fat Sesame Ginger*

Desserts/Snacks

- Fruit 'n Yogurt Parfait (Hold the granola.)
- Apple Dippers with Low-Fat Caramel Dip

BURGER KING

Burgers/Sandwiches

- Tendergrill Chicken Sandwich* without mayo
- Veggie Burger without mayo
- Add Garden Salad to both

Salad

- Tendergrill Chicken Garden Salad

Dressing

- Ken's Fat-Free Ranch Dressing*

Dessert

- Mott's Strawberry-Flavored Applesauce

*high salt content

WENDY'S

Sandwiches

- Ultimate Chicken Grill Sandwich* plus side salad

Salad

- Mandarin Chicken Salad with Roasted Almonds
- Chicken Caesar Salad with Roasted Almonds

Dressings

- Fat-Free French
- Low-Fat Honey Mustard

Other

- Large Chili* with side salad

TACO BELL

- All the Fresco tacos and burritos*

ARBY'S

Sandwiches

- Ham and Swiss Melt*

Salads

- Santa Fe with Grilled Chicken
- Martha's Vineyard Salad

Dressing

- Light Buttermilk Ranch
  (use very sparingly)

*high salt content

KFC

Sandwiches

- Tender Roast Sandwich* without sauce
- Oven-Roasted Twister* without sauce

Chicken

- Chicken breast without skin or breading plus green beans/small corn on the cob

Salads

- Roasted Caesar Salad without dressing and croutons
- Roasted BLT Salad without dressing and croutons

Dressings

- Hidden Valley Golden Italian Light
- Hidden Valley Original Ranch Fat-Free

QUIZNOS

Salads

- Chicken Caesar

Dressings

- Only use fat-free balsamic vinaigrette. The other dressings are a disaster.

Sammies

- All Sammies except Italiano

Subs (small size only)

- All the Turkey subs*—hold the cheese and use light dressing only
- Honey Bourbon Chicken

*high salt content

- Roast Beef and Cheddar
- Honey Ham and Swiss*
- Oven-Roasted Turkey and Cheddar*

PUTTING IT TO THE TEST

Here's how e-Clinic participants stayed in the green while eating out of the house—whether on the road or out for a meal:

"My toughest struggle this week was stadium food. I went to a soccer game. You really are at their mercy; they even check handbags on the way in (they say for security, but you aren't even allowed to bring in your own bottle of water). I had no problem skipping the beer, although usually over the course of the match I would have had two or three. The real problem was not so much craving bad food as the unavailability of anything the least bit healthy. I ended up getting a chicken burrito, begging a fork off another vendor, unwrapping the tortilla, and eating the chicken, beans, tomatoes, and some of the rice. You would think with all the media focus on obesity and healthy eating, someone would open up a salad bar or at least do grilled (as opposed to fried) chicken sandwiches. Maybe there's an opportunity for my second career."—Karen

"Eating out is still the biggest challenge. I went to a birthday party at East Side Mario's [an Italian-American restaurant]. It is almost impossible to find green-light food there, except for the salad, which I ate generously (dressing on the side and used only a little)."—Lynn

*high salt content

"My experience eating regular food at the retreat was really good. I took small amounts of some of the food and left bread and desserts alone. I had cheese sticks, almonds, and apples to eat in between meals, which kept me from being as hungry at mealtime. I allowed myself one treat: homemade cinnamon rolls. I was really surprised when I came home and had lost weight!"—Diane

Beverley, faced with a business trip, took matters into her own hands:

"I was in Toronto for four days last week for meetings and training. Because of time constraints, it was decided that we would start early in the morning and work as long as possible. The decision was also made to eat breakfast and lunch at the training center. I arrived the first morning thinking surely there would be something there I could eat. Wrong. *What they considered breakfast consisted of giant muffins and croissants, tea and coffee—there weren't even any jugs of water. Lunch was a huge tray of sandwiches (all on white buns or croissants) and a few carrot sticks. There was a big salad with the dressing already tossed in. Although it was some kind of oil and vinegar dressing, it was sooo sweet. We were on our own for dinner.*

"I decided I needed to take control over the meals I could. When I returned to the hotel, I requested that a small fridge be delivered to my room. I then went to the grocery store, where I bought Fiber One cereal, skim milk, and fruit, and disposable bowls, cutlery, and bottled water. The next morning I had my breakfast before heading out and felt so much better for it.

"When I arrived at the training center, I spoke with the woman responsible for organizing and asked her to direct me to the person preparing our lunches. I spoke to the nicest 'little' lady from the cafeteria and explained that I can't eat sandwiches laden with butter and mayonnaise, and that I needed a salad not all dressed. She was more than happy to oblige. That afternoon, along with all the sandwiches was a plate of cold meat (not nonfat but okay), cut-up veggies, half a boiled egg, and a big pickle. There was salad with nothing on it and a small container of oil and vinegar with no sugar added. I was happy.

"I will admit that I did have a cocktail after work when everyone met before dinner, but I limited myself to one. I know first-hand that alcohol dismisses willpower. I ate dinner out with the group but was as careful as I could be. This allowed me to go to bed without feeling guilty over what I ate that day. I did this for the rest of my stay.

"Overall, I know there were things I ate that weren't green-light, but I feel really good about how I handled things. Prior to this, I would never have said a word and just ate what was provided for me just so I wouldn't bring attention to myself. But now I realize I am the only one who can control what I eat; I am responsible for myself. I wasn't the least bit embarrassed, and no one said a word about my special requests. It was really no big deal, after all. Best of all, I feel in control and that feels so good."

Wow, that's tremendous, Beverley! Good luck, everyone, taking control of your meals while away from home!

Week 5 Weight: _____

Week 5 Waist: _____

Week 5 Hips: _____

week 5 diary

WEEK 5 OPTIONAL MEAL PLAN

	BREAKFAST	SNACK	LUNCH
MONDAY	Homey Oatmeal (p. 202) with chopped apple	Cranberry Cinnamon Bran Muffin (p. 266)	Open-faced chicken sandwich with lettuce, tomato, and onion, and Basic G.I. Salad (p. 215)
TUESDAY	Mini Breakfast Puffs (p. 206)	Fruit yogurt	G.I. Pasta Salad (p. 224)
WEDNESDAY	Homemade Muesli (p. 203) with skim milk and fruit yogurt	Cranberry Cinnamon Bran Muffin (p. 266)	½ whole wheat pita with canned light tuna, lettuce, tomato, and cucumber, and Basic G.I. Salad (p. 215)
THURSDAY	Homey Oatmeal (p. 202) with blueberries	Small apple and glass of skim milk	Quick and Easy Chicken Noodle Soup (p. 211) and Basic G.I. Salad (p. 215)
FRIDAY	All-Bran Bran Buds (or other high-fiber cereal) with skim milk, peach slices, and sliced almonds	Fruit yogurt	Mixed Bean Salad (p. 222)
SATURDAY	Western Omelet (p. 210)	½ nutrition bar	Greek Salad (p. 218)
SUNDAY	Oatmeal Buttermilk Pancakes (p. 205) with strawberries	Orange and almonds	Tuscan White Bean Soup (p. 213) and Basic G.I. Salad (p. 215)

Note: You are not required to use these weekly meal plans and shopping lists. Feel free to pick and choose and make up your own green-light meals.

SNACK	DINNER	SNACK
Laughing Cow Light cheese with crispbread	Easy-Bake Lasagna (p. 228) and Caesar Salad (p. 216)	Mixed berries tossed in lime juice with fat-free sour cream
Hummus with carrot and celery sticks	G.I. Fish Fillet (p. 237), asparagus, carrots, and new potatoes	Orange and almonds
Babybel Light cheese with crispbread	Chicken Curry (p. 247) and Raita Salad (p. 220)	Apple Pie Cookie (p. 278) and glass of skim milk
Crunchy Chickpeas (p. 271)	Vegetable Crumble (p. 230) and Tabbouleh Salad (p. 221)	½ nutrition bar
Laughing Cow Light cheese with crispbread	Fried Rice with Chicken (p. 246)	Mixed berries tossed in lime juice with fat-free sour cream
Hummus with carrot and celery sticks	Beef and Eggplant Chili (p. 257) and Basic G.I. Salad (p. 215)	Apple Pie Cookie (p. 278) and glass of skim milk
Babybel Light cheese with crispbread	Pork Medallions Dijon (p. 261), green beans, carrots, and new potatoes	Piece of Plum Crumble (p. 275)

grocery list for WEEK 5

These ingredients correspond with the recipes in this week's meal plan. Be sure that your basic pantry is well-stocked—refer to the list on pages 46–47.

produce

- ☐ asparagus
- ☐ bean sprouts
- ☐ eggplant
- ☐ kale
- ☐ leeks
- ☐ iceberg lettuce
- ☐ romaine lettuce
- ☐ prune plums
- ☐ sweet potatoes
- ☐ fresh sage
- ☐ baby spinach
- ☐ fresh tarragon
- ☐ fresh thyme
- ☐ firm tofu
- ☐ zucchini

meat, poultry, and fish

- ☐ extra-lean ground beef
- ☐ pork tenderloins
- ☐ Canadian bacon
- ☐ skinless, boneless chicken breasts
- ☐ fish fillets, such as salmon or trout

dairy and deli

- ☐ low-fat cheddar cheese
- ☐ part-skim mozzarella cheese

pastas

- ☐ whole wheat lasagna
- ☐ whole wheat rotini or penne

miscellaneous

- ☐ dried cranberries
- ☐ raisins
- ☐ flax seeds
- ☐ sesame seeds
- ☐ mixed nuts
- ☐ ground cardamom
- ☐ curry powder
- ☐ kalamata olives
- ☐ low-fat tomato pasta sauce
- ☐ light tomato sauce with no added sugar

week 6:

Unrealistic Expectations

THIS WEEK I WOULD LIKE TO ADDRESS THE CRITICAL ISSUE OF unrealistic expectations. Unfortunately, in this instant gratification society, we tend to want immediate results. Even though it took us years to gain the weight we currently have, we expect to lose it right away. But you can't address a long-term problem like being overweight with a short-term solution. Taking your food intake to extremes by skipping snacks and cutting calories to a dangerously low level just won't work. Slow, steady weight loss is the only healthy and clinically proven way to lose weight permanently. This is why you need a weight-loss plan you can live with for the long haul, which is what the G.I. Diet is all about.

One pound a week is the average that most people lose, and it is certainly nothing to sniff at. (Have you ever seen a pound of fat? It's a substantial amount!) And yet look at some of the comments I received from e-Clinic participants as they found their weight loss slowing from its initial surge:

> *"Disappointed with my week of 'progress.' I stuck to the program pretty well, I even cut back on bread when I wasn't losing at the first of the week. Still only lost one pound."*
>
> —Diane

"Feeling disappointed at the small weight loss this week and the little or no change in measurements. I have gone over my meals for the past week to see if there is something I might have done better."

—Kathy, who lost 2 pounds in one week

"Small weight loss. . . . I'll need to get some exercise to start burning off more weight."

—Ross, who lost 3 pounds in one week

"Thought maybe I would have lost a little more weight, but patience has never been a virtue for me."

—another Kathy, who lost 4 pounds in one week

One, 2, 3, even 4 pounds of weight gone! All of these people should be feeling happy about their weight loss and proud of their achievements. How unfortunate that they aren't giving themselves the pat on the back that they so well deserve. Impatience and disappointment are dangerous: They can derail you from the healthy track you're on and make you want to give up. Just read the following letter from Pat:

"I am really disappointed with myself, as I have only lost one pound this week. I really want the weight to come off faster than it is. . . . I have to tell you, this past Wednesday, midafternoon, I started thinking that I was going to pack this program in. I was thinking again about how the weight wasn't coming off fast enough. But I stopped myself, and asked myself, what really is going on here? Was I hungry, tired, or thirsty? I came to the revelation that I was tired

and really thirsty. Once I stopped and took a rest and had something to drink, I got refocused. I knew in my heart that quitting wasn't what I wanted to do."

It's great that Pat was able to refocus and stick with the program. She had been losing an average of over 1 pound per week, and at that rate she would be reaching her target weight in only nine months—less than a year! In that time she could be at her ideal weight, wearing the clothes she wanted and enjoying her renewed energy and improved health! When you consider the number of years it took to put on the weight, nine months is certainly not an unreasonable time frame. Furthermore, when you are on the G.I. Diet, you know that you are eating in a healthy and nutritious way that is benefiting your body while you reduce. An average of 1 pound per week is right on target.

Yes, there are instances where people have lost 3 to 4 pounds per week, or even more, but frequently they then hit a plateau and their weight loss averages out to a more normal level. It all depends upon many factors, including your metabolism, the amount of weight you have to lose, and the degree to which you stick to the green-light way of eating.

Tammy, one of the e-Clinic participants, found out firsthand that if you lose too much too fast, there's more that happens than just weight loss:

"This last week I am very impressed with my weight loss, but I have been feeling really foggy. I have vertigo and it has been a very bad week for it. I had to leave work early on Friday due to dizziness. I still feel really foggy today. Do you think that it is due to the diet?"

Tammy had been losing an average of 3 pounds per week for six weeks, and I was concerned that she was overdoing things. I suggested she check that her portion sizes were in line with my recommendations and that she was eating her regular three meals and three snacks per day. I also asked her to see her doctor in case there was some other health issue that needed to be addressed.

To end on a positive note, here's a note I received from Jenny, for whom a pound a week was an occasion to celebrate:

> *"One pound a week for me is really good compared to what I was doing on Weight Watchers (which was about 0.2 pounds a week—very frustrating!)."*

Week 6 Weight: _____

Week 6 Waist: _____

Week 6 Hips: _____

week 6 diary

_____

_____

_____

_____

_____

_____

_____

_____

_____

WEEK 6 OPTIONAL MEAL PLAN

	BREAKFAST	SNACK	LUNCH
MONDAY	Homey Oatmeal (p. 202) with chopped apple	Carrot Muffin (p. 267)	Open-faced lean deli ham sandwich with lettuce, tomato, red pepper, and grainy mustard, and Basic G.I. Salad (p. 215)
TUESDAY	Mini Breakfast Puffs (p. 206)	Fruit yogurt	Waldorf Chicken and Rice Salad (p. 226)
WEDNESDAY	Homemade Muesli (p. 203) with skim milk and fruit yogurt	Carrot Muffin (p. 267)	Cottage cheese with apple and grapes, and Basic G.I. Salad (p. 215)
THURSDAY	Homey Oatmeal (p. 202) with blueberries	Small apple and glass of skim milk	Minestrone (p. 212) and Basic G.I. Salad (p. 215)
FRIDAY	All-Bran Bran Buds (or other high-fiber cereal) with skim milk, peach slices, and sliced almonds	Fruit yogurt	½ whole wheat pita with deli turkey, lettuce, tomato, and cucumber, and Basic G.I. Salad (p. 215)
SATURDAY	Italian Omelet (p. 208)	½ nutrition bar	Crab Salad in Tomato Shells (p. 225)
SUNDAY	Cinnamon French Toast (p. 204) with Canadian bacon	Orange and almonds	Ham and Lentil Soup (p. 214) and Basic G.I. Salad (p. 215)

Note: You are not required to use these weekly meal plans and shopping lists. Feel free to pick and choose and make up your own green-light meals.

SNACK	DINNER	SNACK
Laughing Cow Light cheese with crispbread	Fettuccine Primavera (p. 227) and Caesar Salad (p. 216)	Mixed berries tossed in lime juice with fat-free sour cream
Hummus with carrot and celery sticks	Ginger-Wasabi Halibut (p. 240), Cold Noodle Salad with Cucumber and Sesame (p. 223), snow peas and carrots	Orange and almonds
Babybel Light cheese with crispbread	Chicken Tarragon with Mushrooms (p. 245), broccoli, and basmati rice	Pecan Brownie (p. 280) and glass of skim milk
Crunchy Chickpeas (p. 271)	Meat Loaf (p. 259), green beans, carrots, and new potatoes	½ nutrition bar
Laughing Cow Light cheese with crispbread	Bean and Onion Pizza (p. 234)	Mixed berries tossed in lime juice with fat-free sour cream
Hummus with carrot and celery sticks	Grilled Tuna with Chimichurri Sauce (p. 241), asparagus, and new potatoes	Pecan Brownie (p. 280) and glass of skim milk
Babybel Light cheese with crispbread	Orange Chicken with Almonds (p. 250), green beans, and basmati rice	Slice of Apple Raspberry Coffee Cake (p. 272)

grocery list for WEEK 6

These ingredients correspond with the recipes in this week's meal plan. Be sure that your basic pantry is well-stocked—refer to the list on pages 46–47.

produce

- ☐ asparagus
- ☐ fresh basil
- ☐ fresh cilantro
- ☐ fresh ginger
- ☐ grapes
- ☐ raspberries
- ☐ romaine lettuce
- ☐ snow peas
- ☐ baby spinach
- ☐ firm tofu
- ☐ yellow summer squash
- ☐ large beefsteak tomatoes

meat, poultry, and fish

- ☐ extra-lean ground beef
- ☐ Canadian bacon
- ☐ skinless, boneless chicken breasts
- ☐ canned crab
- ☐ halibut fillets
- ☐ tuna steaks, ½ inch thick

dairy and deli

- ☐ part-skim mozzarella cheese
- ☐ low-fat, low-sugar buttermilk salad dressing
- ☐ lean deli ham
- ☐ lean deli turkey

pastas

- ☐ whole wheat capellini or spaghettini
- ☐ whole wheat fettuccine or linguine

miscellaneous

- ☐ active dry yeast
- ☐ raisins
- ☐ sun-dried tomatoes
- ☐ flax seeds
- ☐ sesame seeds
- ☐ pecans
- ☐ walnuts
- ☐ wasabi powder
- ☐ dried tarragon
- ☐ low-fat tomato pasta sauce
- ☐ mirin or sweet sherry
- ☐ tomato juice
- ☐ vegetable cocktail juice

week 7:

Emotional Eating

THIS WEEK WE COVER THE QUESTION OF EMOTIONAL EATING, frequently described as "using food for comfort."

I have asked my wife, Dr. Ruth Gallop, who is Professor Emeritus at the University of Toronto, to write this section because one of her specialties is childhood trauma and how that plays out in adult life. This has given her considerable insight into the role food plays in helping people deal with their emotional issues. We realize that this is a very large topic but hope to provide you with some guidance. Here are Ruth's thoughts.

We all eat for comfort to a lesser or greater extent. When we are sick, many of us have favorite foods—often foods from our childhood. There are foods we eat rarely and foods we could eat every day—often foods that make us feel good or satiated.

When we have reasonably balanced lives, food plays an important but not dominant role. When our lives are out of balance and we don't feel good about certain aspects of them, food can take over. When we don't feel good about ourselves, food can be a powerful and damaging force. This is particularly true for women, because our society is fixated on how we should look. Putting aside all the health reasons for being at a "normal" weight, there is also the fact that our society just doesn't approve of fat people. And more important, fat people often don't approve of themselves.

Eating to feel better is usually preceded by negative feelings. For some people these may include sadness, loneliness, or even a sense of boredom. For others they can be more in the range of anger, irritability, or high stress. These feelings can lead to a vicious eating cycle that goes something like this:

I feel angry/bored/sad/bad about myself.
I eat.
I experience a brief blood sugar high and feel better.
I experience a blood sugar crash and feel terrible.
I feel bad about myself for eating, for failing.
So I eat to feel better . . .
And around I go.

In many situations the original reasons for feeling bad about oneself or getting angry, overwhelmed, or disappointed may have origins in childhood, but overeating, negative body image, and low self-esteem are the present consequence. We do not usually make a conscious link between past events and current behavior. For example, when we were children, parental approval and love may have been connected with food via treats or eating all that was put in front of us. Or we may have been punished—something we might have interpreted as love being withdrawn—if we didn't eat our vegetables. And so eating becomes connected with trying to recapture that good feeling of being loved. Although we might be unaware of these motives or psychological reasons for the behavior, we have been engaging in it for so long that we don't question this part of our food and eating habits.

Rick's mother cannot bear to see food left unfinished on the plate, regardless of whether a person is still hungry. At ninety-seven years of age, she still says "I do like to see a clean plate" when all the food on the table has disappeared. I have learned to deal with this learned behavior—a behavior that earned Rick love and approval from his mother when he was a child—by never putting excess food on the table at mealtimes, trying to plate dishes prior to serving them, and not leaving bowls of food out on the table. Otherwise, Rick's impulse will be to finish the food, and he will unconsciously graze.

How do you change eating behaviors that you learned as a child? You have already taken the most important step: removing all red-light food from the house and making a conscious decision to eat only green-light foods! Make sure you reward yourself for this accomplishment—for instance a new lipstick, tickets to a sports event or the theater, a fashion magazine for that new wardrobe—just make sure it isn't a red-light food!

The second step is to become conscious of your eating habits. For example, when you walk in the front door, is your first stop the fridge or snack cupboard? When you have had a bad day at work or the kids have been a hassle, do you deal with it by eating something sweet or high-fat? When you feel bored and have nothing structured to do, is food the first thing you think of? Are you unable to watch TV without snacking, so large amounts of food pass into your mouth without your realizing it?

Most evenings, I have one piece of dark chocolate if I am watching TV. The other night I realized I was in the middle of eating a second piece, with no memory of reaching down and picking it up! For situations like these, I've found it helps to take a day or two to jot down your eating patterns, noting when automatic behaviors take over and when it is most difficult for you to avoid eating in excess. You'll soon begin to recognize your "at-risk" situations. If food comforts you when you're stressed or compensates for setting unrealistic expectations for yourself, such as getting all the errands done, cooking all the meals, and doing all the child care, you'll start to recognize your patterns and can then consider alternative ways to cope—for example, sharing your tasks with others.

Some emotional eating habits to watch out for include:

- **Grazing.** This is a well-established teenage habit that many people don't grow out of. If you cannot pass a fridge without opening it, grazing is a habit for you.

- **Eating when stressed, angry, irritable, tired, or frustrated.**
- **Eating when sad, bored, or lonely.**
- **Eating too quickly.** Never gobble your food. Remember, it takes twenty to thirty minutes for the stomach to tell the brain that it is full.
- **Eating unconsciously.** Never eat from large packages of food. Instead, put the small portion you plan to eat in a bowl or on a plate, and put the package away.
- **Eating too-large portions.** Thanks to fast-food and family restaurants, many portion sizes have doubled in recent years, and we have brought this "portion distortion" into our homes. Be aware of how much you serve yourself at home.
- **Always eating during a social activity.** This includes sports events, visits with family, or chats with friends. Social events don't need to revolve around food.

Once you have recognized your own unhealthy eating behaviors, change them gradually by modifying one behavior at a time. For example, if you usually walk in the front door and immediately go to the fridge to get a snack, consider it one of your G.I. Diet snack times and make sure that you have a green-light snack ready. If you usually eat while watching television in the evenings, try to think of alternate ways to keep your hands busy. How about putting together a photo album, working a jigsaw puzzle, or even ironing while watching your favorite shows? Or are there things you could do instead of watching TV altogether, like going for a walk, doing a crossword puzzle, taking a class to learn more about a hobby, or even having a hot bath?

Substituting pleasurable activities for those times when we eat unconsciously or emotionally helps to break the vicious cycle I have described above. To start the process, write out a list of substitute activities you enjoy.

Substitute Activities List

1. _____
2. _____
3. _____
4. _____
5. _____

This list will be an important tool to help break those bad eating habits. Refer to it until you feel sure that your new behaviors and eating patterns are your new habits. And don't beat yourself up if you slip—it happens to all of us. Just get back on the wagon. You deserve a pat on the back for your determination to stay on this program, so be sure to reward yourself for your small triumphs—go to a show or game, or buy some flowers or a new CD.

One final thought: Just as your parents' behavior may have influenced your eating behaviors, so in turn your current eating behaviors will affect your children. The following comments from Kathy illustrate this point:

> *"I think more now about what I am going to eat and why, especially if I'm out. I realize now what a lot of junk we feed ourselves. I wish that parents of young children would recognize this and take action, because they don't truly understand (and can't unless they have been there and lived it themselves) the impact that being overweight will have on their child emotionally, psychologically, and physically, and the social stigma they will face."*

Good advice from Ruth! Emotional eating is a subject that resonated with my e-Clinic participants, many of whom have struggled with their weight since childhood.

"I had some emotional eating this week. On Tuesday, my doctor told me my X-rays were clear for pneumonia, but there were spots in the lower lungs. That night I had a steak and some red wine. I figured if I had lung cancer I'd lose weight anyway, so what the hell? Had a CT scan on Wednesday and on Friday found out the spots were scars from previous bouts of bronchitis/pneumonia. That led to a celebratory glass of wine (or two) with dinner. I'm back on track now, but this has been a roller-coaster week."—Karen

"I do recognize that for the past four years as a single parent I have often chosen to eat without any sensation of hunger in an effort to deal with (maybe avoid dealing with) being on my own, the isolation of single parenting, and my disappointment in myself for being in this situation, or just generally feeling sorry for myself at times and not wanting to deny myself a 'treat.' I do recognize that the emotional aspect of my situation has only been made worse by my feelings of upset with myself for being so heavy, and that I have to work hard to reward and console myself in different ways, to build in treats that are not edible."—Bernadette

"I have gained two pounds this week. Disappointed and angry with myself definitely. I can only say that this is a result of emotional eating this week. My stress level at work was at a high level. . . . In addition to this, I have been having a lot of dreams of my deceased parents. . . . All I can say is, 'lesson learned,' and now another week begins and I

must get back on track because losing the weight is extremely important to me. . . . I didn't realize until I started this program how much of an emotional eater I am."—Pat

"I've been through a lot in the past few years, and I know I gained all the extra weight in some effort to 'protect' myself. I am trying to learn to love myself in ways that do not involve reaching for food as a means of consoling myself. I have a long way to go, but I have the basic tools. The stronger I get financially and emotionally, the more I care about my health and appearance."—Nancy

Keep in mind that as you lose weight, you will begin to feel better not only physically but also psychologically. Being successful will improve your self-esteem. Feeling better about how you look is the best reinforcement for holding back on red-light foods and breaking those bad eating habits. You will notice your body changing, and others will, too. As you start to experience success in permanent weight reduction, you will think of yourself as successful. As a reader once said, "I no longer hide behind a tree every time a camera comes out." You may find you feel safe enough to come out into the world. Let people compliment you.

Week 7 Weight: _____

Week 7 Waist: _____

Week 7 Hips: _____

week 7 diary

WEEK 7 OPTIONAL MEAL PLAN

	BREAKFAST	SNACK	LUNCH
MONDAY	Homey Oatmeal (p. 202) with chopped apple	Apple Bran Muffin (p. 264)	Open-faced chicken sandwich with lettuce, tomato, and onion, and Basic G.I. Salad (p. 215)
TUESDAY	Mini Breakfast Puffs (p. 206)	Fruit yogurt	G.I. Pasta Salad (p. 224)
WEDNESDAY	Homemade Muesli (p. 203) with skim milk and fruit yogurt	Apple Bran Muffin (p. 264)	½ whole wheat pita with canned light tuna, lettuce, tomato, and cucumber, and Basic G.I. Salad (p. 215)
THURSDAY	Homey Oatmeal (p. 202) with blueberries	Small apple and glass of skim milk	Quick and Easy Chicken Noodle Soup (p. 211) and Basic G.I. Salad (p. 215)
FRIDAY	All-Bran Bran Buds (or other high-fiber cereal) with skim milk, peach slices, and sliced almonds	Fruit yogurt	Mixed Bean Salad (p. 222)
SATURDAY	Vegetarian Omelet (p. 209)	½ nutrition bar	Greek Salad (p. 218)
SUNDAY	Oatmeal Buttermilk Pancakes (p. 205) with strawberries	Orange and almonds	Tuscan White Bean Soup (p. 213) and Basic G.I. Salad (p. 215)

Note: You are not required to use these weekly meal plans and shopping lists. Feel free to pick and choose and make up your own green-light meals.

SNACK	DINNER	SNACK
Laughing Cow Light cheese with crispbread	Rigatoni with Mini Meatballs (p. 254) and Caesar Salad (p. 216)	Mixed berries tossed in lime juice with fat-free sour cream
Hummus with carrot and celery sticks	Citrus-Poached Haddock (p. 239), green beans, and new potatoes	Orange and almonds
Babybel Light cheese with crispbread	Chicken Jambalaya (p. 256) and broccoli	Creamy Lemon Square (p. 279), and glass of skim milk
Crunchy Chickpeas (p. 271)	Barley Risotto with Leeks, Lemon, and Peas (p. 236), and Tabbouleh Salad (p. 221)	½ nutrition bar
Laughing Cow Light cheese with crispbread	Thai Red Curry Shrimp Pasta (p. 244)	Mixed berries tossed in lime juice with fat-free sour cream
Hummus with carrot and celery sticks	Zesty Barbecued Chicken (p. 252), Tangy Red and Green Coleslaw (p. 219), and new potatoes	Creamy Lemon Square (p. 279) and glass of skim milk
Babybel Light cheese with crispbread	Pork Tenderloin with Apple Compote (p. 260), brussels sprouts, carrots, and new potatoes	Piece of Berry Crumble (p. 274)

grocery list for WEEK 7

These ingredients correspond with the recipes in this week's meal plan. Be sure that your basic pantry is well-stocked—refer to the list on pages 46–47.

produce

- ☐ brussels sprouts
- ☐ cabbage, both green and red
- ☐ fresh cilantro
- ☐ eggplant
- ☐ kale
- ☐ leeks
- ☐ iceberg lettuce
- ☐ romaine lettuce
- ☐ fresh mint
- ☐ fresh rosemary
- ☐ fresh sage
- ☐ fresh thyme
- ☐ zucchini

meat, poultry, and fish

- ☐ pork tenderloin
- ☐ skinless, boneless chicken breasts
- ☐ lean ground chicken or turkey
- ☐ haddock fillets
- ☐ large raw shrimp

dairy and deli

- ☐ low-fat cheddar cheese

pastas

- ☐ whole wheat macaroni or small shells
- ☐ whole wheat rigatoni
- ☐ whole wheat rotini or penne
- ☐ whole wheat spaghettini or linguine

miscellaneous

- ☐ dried currants
- ☐ ground almonds
- ☐ pecans
- ☐ flax seeds
- ☐ celery seeds
- ☐ ground cloves
- ☐ dried sage
- ☐ bay leaves
- ☐ kalamata olives
- ☐ Thai red curry paste
- ☐ light tomato sauce with no added sugar
- ☐ frozen apple juice concentrate
- ☐ unsweetened apple juice
- ☐ unsweetened orange juice

week 8:

Reaching a Plateau

WHEN YOU'RE RIGOROUSLY ADHERING TO THE GREEN-LIGHT way and have been steadily losing weight for many successive weeks, it's difficult to accept that the weight loss can suddenly stall. Unfair as it may be, it is inevitable. Weight loss never occurs in a straight line, but always in a series of steps or plateaus, as all of our e-Clinic participants discovered at one point or another:

> *"Battling a tough weekly result. I'm a little baffled at my lack of weight loss this week, and due to the results I had a bout of emotional eating with a box of doughnut holes. I find it really frustrating (and I've been here before) to do a total 180 on my eating and not have any weight come off."*—Sandra
>
> *"Well, I have found a plateau, but since I knew it was out there waiting for me and this is a marathon not a sprint, I'm okay with it—after a few moments of 'black cloud.' As long as things keep moving forward . . ."*—Ross
>
> *"I am totally surprised and very disappointed. This week I made sure that I ate only green, knowing that I had two dinners out for my birthday. I even went online and checked*

the menus at both places so I could go in knowing exactly what I was going to have and not be tempted by everything else. I skipped the bread basket, the desserts, had grilled chicken and salad with vinaigrette dressing at one place, and grilled salmon, fresh beans and baby carrots, and salad with vinaigrette dressing on my birthday. The only thing I did have was a small glass of wine. No cake, didn't eat one of my favorite cookies that were bought by one of the girls I ride in with on the bus, since we couldn't have a cake, she said. I was so pleased with myself—that was until I stepped on the scale this morning and it showed the 1.5-pound gain and no change in measurements. I just don't understand. I'm at a loss, frustrated, and very disappointed."—Kathy

Many factors show up on the scale: stress, water retention, hormonal shifts, change in exercise schedules, even seasonality. The body tends to naturally want to put on weight for winter and lose a bit for summer due to the feast-and-famine cycles from deep in our ancestral past. Estrogen levels in particular can influence how much water you retain, which is why women experience sudden short-term changes in weight, especially before a period—and even more so during menopause.

For many reasons, your weight can fluctuate significantly even day to day. This is why I suggest you restrict your weigh-in to once a week—you'll avoid the disappointment of these short-term aberrations and focus on your long-term success. Just keep on the green-light track and the weight will continue to come off. Some e-Clinic participants also wondered why they sometimes seemed to be losing inches but not pounds, and sometimes pounds but not inches. Remember, everyone is different, and weight loss doesn't ever happen in a straight line; eventually both the inches and the pounds will come off—guaranteed!

Diet and Menopause

Menopause, which can go on for up to ten years, can impact a woman's weight in two ways. First, estrogen levels decrease, causing erratic swings in water retention and blood sugar levels. When your blood sugar levels drop, your brain calls for more sugar, making you want to reach out for those red-light foods, which will temporarily give you a boost and make you feel better in the short term. The sugar high, however, will cause your insulin to kick in, quickly bringing your blood sugar levels down to another low. We know all about this relentless cycle. That's why it's so important to eat only green-light foods, because they will help stabilize your blood sugar and mood. Second, menopause will slow your metabolic rate, or the rate at which your body burns calories. As you know, to lose weight you have to use up more calories than your body takes in. So if you are burning fewer calories, your rate of weight loss will slow. This is why it can be more of a challenge to lose weight during menopause.

So don't let an irregularity on the scale get you down. Though nothing is quite as frustrating as hitting a weight-loss plateau, if you hang in there—and don't use food to console yourself—you will get past it and continue toward your weight-loss target. Here is how some e-Clinic participants tried to focus on the positive as they encountered plateaus:

> *"I thought I had done well this week and was sure I had a good loss. . . . It was disappointing when the scale said I'd lost only half a pound and virtually nothing in inches. I can't believe that with the amount of weight I have to lose my body would be considering plateauing yet! I know I feel*

good and that I made good decisions this week, but I just didn't see any rewards. I don't know how much my monthly cycle plays in this, as I was on all week. . . . Oh well, as they say, Rome wasn't built in a day, and I'm not going to lose all this weight in a day, a month, or even a year (sounds daunting!)."—Kathy

"I like to weigh myself daily because I feel it keeps me on track. It does not discourage me. I have always done it that way. The only exception I make is if I know I had a really bad day, then I will wait a day to weigh myself. But I have noticed since my weight has been going down that it will be down for a few days then pop back up to the older weight and then a few days later back down it will go. The encouraging part is that each time it goes up it is not as far as the time before."—Diane

"No weight loss this week, but my other numbers (measurements) are down. . . . At this point I have lost 15 pounds, 4.5 inches from waist, and 4.5 inches from hips, and my BMI is down from 38.4 to 36. I know the scale is one measurement to use, but that's only one number. I am also looking at my other numbers, and for me, using these other numbers helps keep me from being disappointed when the scale does not move."—Jenny

Week 8 Weight: _____

Week 8 Waist: _____

Week 8 Hips: _____

week 8 diary

WEEK 8 OPTIONAL MEAL PLAN

	BREAKFAST	SNACK	LUNCH
MONDAY	Homey Oatmeal (p. 202) with chopped apple	Whole Wheat Fruit Scone (p. 269)	Open-faced lean deli ham sandwich with lettuce, tomato, red pepper, and grainy mustard, and Basic G.I. Salad (p. 215)
TUESDAY	Mini Breakfast Puffs (p. 206)	Fruit yogurt	Waldorf Chicken and Rice Salad (p. 226)
WEDNESDAY	Homemade Muesli (p. 203) with skim milk and fruit yogurt	Whole Wheat Fruit Scone (p. 269)	Cottage cheese with apple and grapes, and Basic G.I. Salad (p. 215)
THURSDAY	Homey Oatmeal (p. 202) with blueberries	Small apple and glass of skim milk	Minestrone (p. 212) and Basic G.I. Salad (p. 215)
FRIDAY	All-Bran Bran Buds (or other high-fiber cereal) with skim milk, peach slices, and sliced almonds	Fruit yogurt	½ whole wheat pita with deli turkey, lettuce, tomato, and cucumber, and Basic G.I. Salad (p. 215)
SATURDAY	Canadian Bacon Omelet (p. 207)	½ nutrition bar	Crab Salad in Tomato Shells (p. 225)
SUNDAY	Cinnamon French Toast (p. 204) with Canadian bacon	Orange and almonds	Ham and Lentil Soup (p. 214) and Basic G.I. Salad (p. 215)

Note: You are not required to use these weekly meal plans and shopping lists. Feel free to pick and choose and make up your own green-light meals.

SNACK	DINNER	SNACK
Laughing Cow Light cheese with crispbread	Salmon Pasta (p. 238)	Mixed berries tossed in lime juice with fat-free sour cream
Hummus with carrot and celery sticks	Pan-Seared Whitefish with Mandarin Salsa (p. 242), broccoli, and basmati rice	Orange and almonds
Babybel Light cheese with crispbread	Chicken Schnitzel (p. 248), green beans, carrots, and new potatoes	Slice of Strawberry Tea Bread (p. 270) and glass of skim milk
Crunchy Chickpeas (p. 271)	Mushroom Gravy Pork Chops (p. 263), asparagus, and basmati rice	½ nutrition bar
Laughing Cow Light cheese with crispbread	Horseradish Burgers (p. 258) and Tabbouleh Salad (p. 221)	Mixed berries tossed in lime juice with fat-free sour cream
Hummus with carrot and celery sticks	Vegetarian Moussaka (p. 232) and basmati rice	Slice of Strawberry Tea Bread (p. 270) and glass of skim milk
Babybel Light cheese with crispbread	Spicy Roast Chicken with Tomatoes and Tarragon (p. 249), green beans, and basmati rice	Slice of One-Bowl Chocolate Cake (p. 276)

grocery list for WEEK 8

These ingredients correspond with the recipes in this week's meal plan. Be sure that your basic pantry is well-stocked—refer to the list on pages 46–47.

produce

- ☐ alfalfa sprouts (optional)
- ☐ asparagus
- ☐ fresh basil
- ☐ fresh cilantro
- ☐ eggplant
- ☐ grapes
- ☐ fresh mint
- ☐ baby spinach
- ☐ fresh tarragon
- ☐ large beefsteak tomatoes
- ☐ cherry or grape tomatoes

meat, poultry, and fish

- ☐ extra-lean ground beef
- ☐ boneless pork loin chops
- ☐ Canadian bacon
- ☐ skinless, boneless chicken breasts
- ☐ canned crab
- ☐ salmon fillet
- ☐ whitefish fillets

dairy and deli

- ☐ low-fat, low-sugar buttermilk salad dressing
- ☐ light herb and garlic cream cheese
- ☐ lean deli ham
- ☐ lean deli turkey

pastas

- ☐ whole wheat macaroni or small shells

miscellaneous

- ☐ dried apricots
- ☐ sun-dried tomatoes
- ☐ dried basil
- ☐ Italian herb seasoning
- ☐ prepared horseradish
- ☐ pecans
- ☐ walnuts
- ☐ unsweetened apple juice
- ☐ unsweetened orange juice
- ☐ whole wheat bread crumbs
- ☐ whole wheat hamburger buns

week 9:

Staying Motivated

WE ARE NOW NEARLY TWO THIRDS OF THE WAY THROUGH THE first thirteen weeks of the G.I. Diet—it's a great time to reflect on your progress to date and what still needs to be done to keep your motivation high.

Over their first eight weeks, e-Clinic participants reported a wide range of results. Some took to the green-light way of eating like the proverbial duck to water, whereas others struggled to make the transition from their red-light habits. Most of the problems participants experienced had nothing to do with the Diet specifically, but with stress, emotions, work and home pressures, and unrelated health issues. The common thread, however, was that they were all determined to get that weight devil off their backs.

This week, I want to discuss keeping determination strong. You wouldn't be human if you didn't feel your resolve starting to waver from time to time. When it does, there are a number of things you can do to encourage yourself to keep going:

1. Remember your initial reasons. Reread your reasons for wanting to lose weight (page 55). Remember why it was so important to you to slim down when you started this journey, and why you need to persevere.

2. Use physical reminders of your goal. Keep a picture of an outfit you're going to buy when you reach your goal or a photograph of a thinner you where you will see it every day:

"A picture or two of yourself really helps, I think. Although you know you are overweight, your mental picture of yourself is not of an overweight person. I can only speak for myself here. Once I saw some pictures of how I really looked, how I looked to others, and that was a big help in motivating me."—Ross

"I am using my beautiful red leather coat to motivate me. Last winter, when I went to put it on, it was about 2 inches too small. I was not able to close the zipper. Now, when I put the coat on, I am able to zip it up. Tight, yes, but I know that I have made progress. What an incredible feeling. . . . I am determined to wear the coat this winter."—Pat

"I had reached the point where I had to buy clothing in the Big Women's section of a shop. I was determined that that was not going to happen again. I dropped almost 25 pounds, and with my clothes falling off of me, I no longer felt that strain on my waistband if I overindulged. So, I've done two things: (1) I've gone into the closet and found even smaller clothes than the ones that now fit. The discomfort is a reminder that I've got a long way to go. And (2) I recently went shopping for new clothes. Instead of trying on and buying size 16 (which I am now down to) I found the prettiest things I could find in 12 and 14 which were not available in my size. I tried them on in the dressing room to get an idea of how much more I have to do before I can just walk into a shop and pick up anything I like."—Karen

3. Keep in mind how far you've come. Compare yourself now to where you were before you started the Diet. How much weight have you lost? How much better do your clothes fit? How have your energy level and health improved? What can you do now that you couldn't do before? Going back to your old eating habits won't seem so tempting when you think how it will undermine all the good things that weight loss has brought you so far.

> *"I realized this morning that I am no longer experiencing heartburn at night, which is an added bonus."*—Nancy
>
> *"I did notice yesterday when I put on a sweatshirt from last year that it was big. What a great feeling. When I was putting away my summer clothes, I said to myself, 'I won't be using these again.' What a motivator."*—Pat
>
> *"I've officially broken below 260, something I've never accomplished before on any other diet. I'm so excited!"*—J

4. Try the "shopping bag cure." People often don't realize how much a pound actually weighs. Sounds crazy, but when people tell me they've lost "only" 20 pounds, I think back to my wife's reaction to carrying dumbbells up a flight of stairs (see pages 53–54), and ask them to fill a couple of shopping bags with 20 pounds of books and carry them up and down the stairs a few times. Everyone is always glad to put the bags down, and they report that they had no idea how heavy 20 pounds really is!

So the next time you're feeling uninspired, fill a shopping bag (or two) with the amount of books, cans of food, or bottles of water that equals how much weight you've lost over the last eight weeks of the program and carry it up and down a flight of stairs three times. You'll be amazed at what you've lost, and you'll be relieved to put the bag down. You couldn't have put down the weight that was around your waist, hips, and thighs a few weeks ago!

Keep the bag intact, and add more books or cans as you continue to lose weight. It's a wonderful motivator.

"Many years ago, I had lost a lot of weight. When I was at a 20-pound loss, a dear skinny friend said to me, 'Diana, do you realize you have lost the equivalent of a 20-pound bag of potatoes? Just carry that around for a while to see how much you have lost.' I have often thought about that. And yes, I have noticed a big difference in my energy level; going up and down steps is not nearly as hard. My joints do not ache as much and my blood pressure is so much better. And my clothes are also fitting better. So even though I've lost 'only 13 pounds,' I am feeling the effects and do not want to go backwards!"—Diana

"At last, I'm below the dreaded 300—never to be seen again! . . . I didn't think this day would ever arrive. Although 21 pounds doesn't seem like a lot if you look at the whole picture, it was my first target in my journey. . . . It's 21 pounds in the right direction, and when I held 21 pounds of kitty litter in the store I realized it's a lot of weight to be carrying every day—no wonder my knees and back hurt!"—Kathy

5. Get support. Buddy up with others who are trying to lose weight: friends, a spouse, or family members. They will give you a sense of camaraderie and encouragement as you strive toward your goal, and you can turn to them for support when you need it.

"The BEST way to stay motivated is to do the program with someone else. My 'G.I. Jane' group has been a fantastic source of inspiration and motivation. When one of us is down, the others pick us up. When we are all down at the same time, we have a group meeting and rekindle the reasons we are doing all of this."—Lynn

"My friend Kathy is also a part of this program. Part of our weekly chat is to check in with one another on our progress and to provide support. We are good at giving one another praise when it is appropriate and providing words of encouragement, too. We also discuss our accomplishments and challenges. It really helps to have a good buddy system. It makes the journey easier."—Pat

"My kids are young but very supportive, as I have told them I am trying to make better food choices so that I will be healthy for a long time. (They have decided that this means I will be able to babysit when I am a grandma to their kids! They are only six and nine!)"—Bernadette

"The holiday barrage of social events starts this coming Friday night, but I think I have that one under control. I had a long conversation with a male friend and told him what I have been doing, which was a surprise in itself, as I don't normally share that kind of information. But he was thrilled and is so supportive—it really felt good. And he will also be at the Friday event."—Kathy

"I would like to suggest to everyone that they need to find a good friend to be accountable to. Someone to share with. That is one good thing I have done differently this time.

Usually, I do not mention I am dieting to anyone. . . . That way 'when' I fail I don't look like a fool again. This time, I have mentioned it to several people. They are also my inspiration to continue. I know they are watching how I eat and how my clothes fit! I know that I can pick any one of them to be accountable to each week if I feel the need. However, I know that the person I need to be accountable to the most is me! I am the one that will benefit by my sticking to this new eating habit and not anyone else!"—Diane

6. The $10 cure This is a motivator that people often stumble upon by accident. The siren song of a red-light lunch draws you into a fast-food chain, where you order a burger with the works, a large French fries, and a shake. Midafternoon, you feel lethargic, unfocused, lazy, even depressed, and you're wondering what hit you. Well, it started with your high-G.I., high-calorie lunch. This caused your blood sugar levels to rocket, which made you feel really good for a couple of hours. Your body, however, doesn't like high blood sugar levels (called hyperglycemia) and releases insulin to take that sugar out of circulation. Sugar levels drop sharply and you are now feeling the effects of a sugar low (hypoglycemia). Because sugar (glucose) is the body's source of energy, of which up to 40 percent goes to fuel the brain, it's not hard to see why those sugar levels cause this down feeling. You've found out the hard way where straying from the green-light path gets you, and your commitment to the G.I. Diet is renewed.

"When you mentioned in your book how horrible you'd feel eating red-light foods after going on this Diet, you weren't kidding!"—J

I call this the $10 cure because it's the food version of what immigrants (like me) used to call the "$1,000 cure." Whenever a new arrival started to pine for "the old country" after a long, cold winter in Canada, the cure was to get on a plane and go home for a week. All the reasons that originally persuaded the person to emigrate would come crashing back, and the thought of flying back to Canada would begin to look pretty good again.

With food, the cure costs less than $1,000—$10 or so isn't that much to pay at all. But this is a motivator of last resort only; I certainly don't want to encourage people to abuse their bodies and feel awful! If you've been unceasingly pining for red-light foods, however, go out and indulge: Order a high-G.I. meal—perhaps pastrami on a kaiser, large fries, a slice of raisin pie à la mode, and a Coke to wash it down. Your mouth may enjoy it, but I guarantee that a couple of hours later you'll be regretting the deviation!

> *"On the couple days I made poor choices, I definitely noticed a difference in how I felt afterwards: depressed, lethargic, and a bit nauseated. That, combined with the minute weight loss, has encouraged me that I need to avoid any deviations because they have such a trickle-down effect."*—Jenny

Staying motivated is crucial to successful weight loss. It keeps you focused and on the green-light path, and it will get you through the pitfalls you'll encounter. Be sure to use the above strategies as needed—and you probably have a couple of your own that work well, too.

Week 9 Weight: _____

Week 9 Waist: _____

Week 9 Hips: _____

week 9 diary

WEEK 9 OPTIONAL MEAL PLAN

	BREAKFAST	SNACK	LUNCH
MONDAY	Homey Oatmeal (p. 202) with chopped apple	Cranberry Cinnamon Bran Muffin (p. 266)	Open-faced chicken sandwich with lettuce, tomato, and onion, and Basic G.I. Salad (p. 215)
TUESDAY	Mini Breakfast Puffs (p. 206)	Fruit yogurt	G.I. Pasta Salad (p. 224)
WEDNESDAY	Homemade Muesli (p. 203) with skim milk and fruit yogurt	Cranberry Cinnamon Bran Muffin (p. 266)	½ whole wheat pita with canned light tuna, lettuce, tomato, and cucumber, and Basic G.I. Salad (p. 215)
THURSDAY	Homey Oatmeal (p. 202) with blueberries	Small apple and glass of skim milk	Quick and Easy Chicken Noodle Soup (p. 211) and Basic G.I. Salad (p. 215)
FRIDAY	All-Bran Bran Buds (or other high-fiber cereal) with skim milk, peach slices, and sliced almonds	Fruit yogurt	Mixed Bean Salad (p. 222)
SATURDAY	Western Omelet (p. 210)	½ nutrition bar	Greek Salad (p. 218)
SUNDAY	Oatmeal Buttermilk Pancakes (p. 205) with strawberries	Orange and almonds	Tuscan White Bean Soup (p. 213) and Basic G.I. Salad (p. 215)

Note: You are not required to use these weekly meal plans and shopping lists. Feel free to pick and choose and make up your own green-light meals.

SNACK	DINNER	SNACK
Laughing Cow Light cheese with crispbread	Easy-Bake Lasagna (p. 228) and Caesar Salad (p. 216)	Mixed berries tossed in lime juice with fat-free sour cream
Hummus with carrot and celery sticks	G.I. Fish Fillet (p. 237), asparagus, carrots, and new potatoes	Orange and almonds
Babybel Light cheese with crispbread	Chicken Curry (p. 247) and Raita Salad (p. 220)	Apple Pie Cookie (p. 278) and glass of skim milk
Crunchy Chickpeas (p. 271)	Vegetable Crumble (p. 230) and Tabbouleh Salad (p. 221)	½ nutrition bar
Laughing Cow Light cheese with crispbread	Fried Rice with Chicken (p. 246)	Mixed berries tossed in lime juice with fat-free sour cream
Hummus with carrot and celery sticks	Beef and Eggplant Chili (p. 257) and Basic G.I. Salad (p. 215)	Apple Pie Cookie (p. 278) and glass of skim milk
Babybel Light cheese with crispbread	Pork Medallions Dijon (p. 261), green beans, carrots, and new potatoes	Piece of Plum Crumble (p. 275)

grocery list for WEEK 9

These ingredients correspond with the recipes in this week's meal plan. Be sure that your basic pantry is well-stocked—refer to the list on pages 46–47.

produce

- ☐ asparagus
- ☐ bean sprouts
- ☐ eggplant
- ☐ kale
- ☐ leeks
- ☐ iceberg lettuce
- ☐ romaine lettuce
- ☐ fresh mint
- ☐ prune plums
- ☐ sweet potato
- ☐ fresh sage
- ☐ baby spinach
- ☐ fresh tarragon
- ☐ fresh thyme
- ☐ firm tofu
- ☐ zucchini

meat, poultry, and fish

- ☐ extra-lean ground beef
- ☐ pork tenderloins
- ☐ Canadian bacon
- ☐ skinless, boneless chicken breasts
- ☐ fish fillets, such as salmon or trout

dairy and deli

- ☐ low-fat cheddar cheese
- ☐ part-skim mozzarella cheese

pastas

- ☐ whole wheat lasagna
- ☐ whole wheat rotini or penne

miscellaneous

- ☐ dried cranberries
- ☐ raisins
- ☐ sesame seeds
- ☐ flax seeds
- ☐ mixed nuts
- ☐ ground cardamom
- ☐ curry powder
- ☐ kalamata olives
- ☐ light tomato sauce with no added sugar
- ☐ low-fat tomato pasta sauce

week 10:

Your Health—What's at Stake

THIS WEEK'S TOPIC FLOWS FROM LAST WEEK'S DISCUSSION OF motivation, because one of the top motivating factors for losing weight, as we saw in Week 1, is the desire to achieve better health. The connection between being overweight and being at increased risk for certain diseases is well established. Let's look at these risks in turn.

HEART DISEASE AND STROKE

Given that I was the president of the Heart and Stroke Foundation of Ontario for fifteen years, it is hardly surprising that I'm starting with these diseases. There is a more important reason, however: Heart disease and stroke cause 32 percent of North American deaths. Remarkably, this is evidence of progress. When I first joined the foundation, the figure was close to 50 percent.

This is a good news/bad news story. The good news is that advances in surgery, drug therapies, and emergency services have saved many lives. The bad news is that we quadruple our risk of heart disease and stroke if we practice any two of the following lifestyle risk factors: being obese, smoking, having hypertension, or being inactive. That number increases to between eight and twenty times the risk if we adopt three or more of these factors. Though the smoking rate has dropped sharply, we are eating more and exercising less, leading inevitably to a more obese and unhealthy population. And though heart disease, like most cancers, is primarily a disease of old age, nearly half of those who suffer heart attacks are under the age of sixty-five. It has been calculated that if we led even a slightly more moderate lifestyle, we could significantly reduce the carnage from these diseases.

A familiar refrain that I have heard many times is "Why worry? If I have a heart attack, today's medicine will save me." It might well save you from immediate death, but the heart is permanently damaged after an attack—it can't repair itself, because its cells don't reproduce. After a heart attack, the heart has to work harder, but it never can compensate for the damage it sustained. It slowly degenerates under this stress, and patients finally "drown" as blood circulation fails and the lungs fill with liquid. Congestive heart failure is a dreadful way to die, so it's important to make sure you do everything you can to avoid having a heart attack in the first place.

The simple fact is the more overweight you are, the more likely it is that you will suffer a heart attack or stroke. The two key factors that link diet to heart disease and stroke are hypertension (high blood pressure) and cholesterol.

High blood pressure puts more stress on the arterial system, causing it to age and deteriorate more rapidly, and ultimately leads to arterial damage, blood clots, and heart attack or stroke. Excess weight has a major bearing on high blood pressure: One Canadian study found that obese adults aged eighteen to fifty-five had a five to thirteen times greater risk of hypertension. A further study demonstrated that a lower-fat diet coupled with a major increase in fruits and vegetables (eight to ten servings a day) lowered blood pressure. The moral: Lose weight and eat more fruits and vegetables to help reduce your blood pressure levels. In other words, eat the green-light way.

Cholesterol is essential to your body's metabolism. High cholesterol is a problem, however, because it's the key ingredient in the plaque that can build up in your arteries, eventually cutting off the blood supply to your heart (causing heart attack) or your brain (leading to stroke). To make things more complicated, there are two forms of cholesterol: HDL (good) cholesterol and LDL (bad) cholesterol. (Remember it this way: HDL is Heart's Delight Level and LDL is Leads to Death Level.) The idea is to boost the HDL level while lowering the LDL level.

The villain when it comes to high LDL levels is saturated fat, which is usually the sort of fat that is solid at room temperature and is found primarily in meat and whole milk products (think of the white fat and marbling in a raw steak, or a piece of whole-milk cheese). On the other hand, the two other types of fat, polyunsaturated and monounsaturated, not only lower LDL levels but also boost HDL. The moral: Make sure some fat is included in your diet, but make sure it's the right fat (see pages 6–8).

DIABETES

Diabetes is the kissing cousin of heart disease: More people die from heart complications arising from diabetes than from diabetes alone. And diabetes rates are skyrocketing: They are expected to double in the next ten years. The principal causes of the most common form of diabetes, Type 2, are obesity and lack of exercise, and the current epidemic is strongly correlated to the obesity trend. The most dramatic illustration of this link I've heard of appears in demographic studies of Canada's Native Indian population, where in some communities diabetes affects nearly half the adults. Hundreds of years ago, before the Europeans colonized North America, the native population lived in a state of feast or famine. When there was an abundance of food, plant or animal, it was stored in the body as fat. In lean times, such as winter, the body depleted these fat supplies. As a result, their bodies developed a "thrift gene," with those who stored and utilized their food most effectively being the survivors—a classic Darwinian example of survival of the fittest. But in contemporary society, where we've taken away famine and the need to hunt or to harvest food—that is, the necessity of exercise—and replaced it with a trip to the supermarket whenever food is required, the result is inevitable: a massive increase in obesity and, with it, diabetes.

Foods with a low G.I. rating, which release sugar more slowly into the bloodstream, appear to play a major role in helping diabetics control their disease. Thus the G.I. Diet provides an opportunity both to lose weight and to assist in the management of the disease. In its magazine, *Diabetes Dialogue*, the Canadian Diabetes Association selected the G.I. Diet as its diet of choice. Because protein and fat affect a food's G.I. rating, people with diabetes should be particularly careful about eating the right balance of green-light protein, carbohydrates, and fat at every meal and snack, and as with any new diet, they should discuss the program with a doctor or another nutrition professional before beginning. Prevention, however, is far preferable to scrambling to fix things that have gone wrong, so keep going with your green-light program and continue to slim down.

CANCER

There is increasing research evidence that diets high in saturated fat are linked to certain cancers, particularly prostate and colorectal. A 2005 global report by the American Institute for Cancer Research concluded that 30 to 40 percent of cancers are directly linked to dietary choices. Its key recommendation is that individuals should choose a diet that includes a variety of vegetables, fruit, and grains, and is low in saturated fat—in a nutshell, the G.I. Diet.

ALZHEIMER'S DISEASE

As with cancer, there is increasing evidence linking certain dementias, particularly Alzheimer's, with fat intake. A recent U.S. study showed that people who ate a diet high in saturated fat were 2.3 times more likely to develop Alzheimer's disease than those whose diet was low in this kind of fat.

ABDOMINAL FAT AND HEALTH

Although your BMI (see pages 16–17) is a measure of body fat based on your height and weight, it is not necessarily the best guide for assessing your health risk. Where you're storing the fat is the real issue. The results of a 2005 worldwide survey involving 27,000 people showed that people who carried their extra weight around their waists (i.e., had apple-shaped bodies) were at far greater risk of disease than those who carried their weight lower down on their hips (pear-shaped). From the study came this table showing the risk of disease based on weight and waist measurement.

Weight	BMI	Waist: Women less than 35" Men less than 40"	Waist: Women 35" plus Men 40" plus
Normal	18.0–24.9	No risk increase	No risk increase
Overweight	25.0–29.9	Increased risk	High risk
Obese	30.0–39.9	High risk	Very high risk

A "beer belly" is not just extra weight. Rather—and quite surprisingly—it is an active, living part of your body. Once it has formed sufficient mass, abdominal fat behaves like an organ, such as the liver, heart, or kidney, except that instead of contributing to your health, it pumps out a dangerous combination of free fatty acids and proteins. The fact is that abdominal fat has many of the characteristics of a huge tumor. A waist measurement of 35 inches or more for women and 40 inches or more for men puts you in the "High Risk" category for developing heart disease, stroke, hypertension (high blood pressure), and certain types of cancer—breast, uterus, and colon for women, prostate and colon for men.

A further refinement is your waist-to-hip ratio. This is calculated by dividing your waist measurement by your hip measurement. A healthy ratio for women is 0.85 or below, and 0.95 or below for men. If you are a woman with a hip measurement of 42 inches and a waist measurement of 38 inches, your waist-to-hip ratio is 0.90, which puts you at risk. If, however, your hip measurement was still 42 inches but your waist was only 34 inches, your ratio would be an acceptable 0.80.

JOINT DEGENERATION

Finally there is the issue of joint degeneration caused by excessive weight loading. In 2008 *Arthritis Care & Research*, an official journal of the American College of Rheumatology, published a survey of knee and hip replacements performed in the United States between 1997 and 2004. Hip replacements had increased during this time by 48 percent and knee replacements by an amazing 63 percent. A similar Canadian report showed that overweight patients accounted for 87 percent of all knee replacements and 74 percent of all hip replacements. The correlation is straightforward: The more weight that's placed on your joints, the faster they wear out. The slimmer you are, the easier the burden on your joints.

If you want to reduce your risk for these diseases and keep your joints intact, then keep up your green-light diet. I can't think of a better motivator.

Week 10 Weight: _____

Week 10 Waist: _____

Week 10 Hips: _____

week 10 diary

WEEK 10 OPTIONAL MEAL PLAN

	BREAKFAST	SNACK	LUNCH
MONDAY	Homey Oatmeal (p. 202) with chopped apple	Carrot Muffin (p. 267)	Open-faced lean deli ham sandwich with lettuce, tomato, red pepper, and grainy mustard, and Basic G.I. Salad (p. 215)
TUESDAY	Mini Breakfast Puffs (p. 206)	Fruit yogurt	Waldorf Chicken and Rice Salad (p. 226)
WEDNESDAY	Homemade Muesli (p. 203) with skim milk and fruit yogurt	Carrot Muffin (p. 267)	Cottage cheese with apple and grapes, and Basic G.I. Salad (p. 215)
THURSDAY	Homey Oatmeal (p. 202) with blueberries	Small apple and glass of skim milk	Minestrone (p. 212) and Basic G.I. Salad (p. 215)
FRIDAY	All-Bran Bran Buds (or other high-fiber cereal) with skim milk, peach slices, and sliced almonds	Fruit yogurt	½ whole wheat pita with deli turkey, lettuce, tomato, and cucumber, and Basic G.I. Salad (p. 215)
SATURDAY	Italian Omelet (p. 208)	½ nutrition bar	Crab Salad in Tomato Shells (p. 225)
SUNDAY	Cinnamon French Toast (p. 204) with Canadian bacon	Orange and almonds	Ham and Lentil Soup (p. 214) and Basic G.I. Salad (p. 215)

Note: You are not required to use these weekly meal plans and shopping lists. Feel free to pick and choose and make up your own green-light meals.

SNACK	DINNER	SNACK
Laughing Cow Light cheese with crispbread	Fettuccine Primavera (p. 227) and Caesar Salad (p. 216)	Mixed berries tossed in lime juice with fat-free sour cream
Hummus with carrot and celery sticks	Ginger-Wasabi Halibut (p. 240), Cold Noodle Salad with Cucumber and Sesame (p. 223), snow peas and carrots	Orange and almonds
Babybel Light cheese with crispbread	Chicken Tarragon with Mushrooms (p. 245), broccoli, and basmati rice	Pecan Brownie (p. 280) and glass of skim milk
Crunchy Chickpeas (p. 271)	Meat Loaf (p. 259), green beans, carrots, and new potatoes	½ nutrition bar
Laughing Cow Light cheese with crispbread	Bean and Onion Pizza (p. 234)	Mixed berries tossed in lime juice with fat-free sour cream
Hummus with carrot and celery sticks	Grilled Tuna with Chimichurri Sauce (p. 241), asparagus, and new potatoes	Pecan Brownie (p. 280) and glass of skim milk
Babybel Light cheese with crispbread	Orange Chicken with Almonds (p. 250), green beans, and basmati rice	Slice of Apple Raspberry Coffee Cake (p. 272)

grocery list for WEEK 10

These ingredients correspond with the recipes in this week's meal plan. Be sure that your basic pantry is well-stocked—refer to the list on pages 46–47.

produce

- ☐ asparagus
- ☐ fresh basil
- ☐ fresh cilantro
- ☐ fresh ginger
- ☐ grapes
- ☐ raspberries
- ☐ snow peas
- ☐ baby spinach
- ☐ firm tofu
- ☐ large beefsteak tomatoes
- ☐ yellow summer squash

meat, poultry, and fish

- ☐ extra-lean ground beef
- ☐ Canadian bacon
- ☐ skinless, boneless chicken breasts
- ☐ canned crab
- ☐ halibut fillets
- ☐ tuna steaks, ½ inch thick

dairy and deli

- ☐ part-skim mozzarella cheese
- ☐ low-fat, low-sugar buttermilk salad dressing
- ☐ lean deli ham
- ☐ lean deli turkey

pastas

- ☐ whole wheat capellini or spaghettini
- ☐ whole wheat fettuccine or linguine

miscellaneous

- ☐ active dry yeast
- ☐ dried cranberries
- ☐ raisins
- ☐ sun-dried tomatoes
- ☐ wasabi powder
- ☐ sesame seeds
- ☐ pecans
- ☐ walnuts
- ☐ flax seeds
- ☐ dried tarragon
- ☐ mirin or sweet sherry
- ☐ tomato juice
- ☐ vegetable cocktail juice
- ☐ low-fat tomato pasta sauce

week 11:

Holidays, Celebrations, and Special Events

THE MOST DIFFICULT TIME OF YEAR FOR ANYONE TRYING TO lose weight is undoubtedly around the winter holidays. Although it may not actually be the holiday season as you are reading this chapter, the advice here can be applied to any sort of celebratory occasion, such as an anniversary, birthday, wedding, or bar mitzvah. And of course you can always turn to this chapter when you are faced with the challenge of an approaching holiday.

Celebrations like Easter, Passover, Christmas, and Thanksgiving all center around an abundance of food, and much of it is red-light. Many people gain weight as they indulge in the feasts at family get-togethers, office cocktail parties, and neighbors' open houses, but it doesn't have to be this way! You can enjoy all the festivities and still stay mostly in the green. It is probably unrealistic to expect you will lose weight during holiday time, but a reasonable goal should be not to put on any more—after all, you've worked hard to achieve all you have so far, and you don't want to undo it! Here are my suggestions for navigating this dangerous terrain.

THE COCKTAIL PARTY

Never go to a cocktail party hungry, or you are likely to overindulge. Instead, have a small green-light meal or snack before heading out for the evening. A bowl of high-fiber green-light cereal or some leftovers from an earlier green-light meal will do the trick.

Once you arrive at a cocktail party, be sure to get yourself a drink. It's important to always have a glass in your hand at a cocktail party; if you don't, someone will probably pass you one that you haven't chosen—or you'll be looking for nibbles to occupy your empty hands. Club soda with a twist of lime or a diet caffeine-free soft drink are good green-light choices.

If you really would like an alcoholic beverage, bypass the beer and fancy cocktails, which are calorie nightmares, and instead choose a white wine spritzer or a glass of dry red wine. Try to limit yourself to one alcoholic drink, and then switch to club soda. Be sure to consume any alcohol with food to slow the rate at which you metabolize it. Look for green-light snacks to sustain you: for example, mixed raw vegetables, low-fat dips such as hummus and salsa, lean sliced turkey and deli ham, steamed or poached shrimp (not breaded), smoked salmon (hold the crème fraîche), and fruit. Do not station yourself beside the bowls of nuts and olives—they may be green-light, but restricting yourself to a small handful of these snacks will prove difficult.

THE HOLIDAY DINNER

It's easy to make a traditional festive meal green-light with some minor adjustments. Hosting the holiday dinner yourself will obviously give you far greater control over the food served than would going to the home of a friend or family member. As a visitor, however, you can still exert some influence by bringing a green-light side dish or dessert, and by serving yourself only from the green-light foods your host serves.

Compose your plate as you would at home: vegetables on half the plate, rice or pasta on one quarter, and a source of protein on the other quarter. Pass on the rolls and mashed potatoes—have extra vegetables instead. If you wish, you can allow yourself a concession by having a small serving of dessert. If you don't have much of a sweet tooth, you might prefer to have a glass of wine instead. Try not to indulge in both.

Here are some additional guidelines, course by course, for serving a green-light holiday meal at home:

Soup: Start the meal with a delicious homemade green-light soup made with stock, vegetables, and fresh herbs.

Salad: Always serve a large salad with homemade green-light dressing. Make it more festive by adding toasted pecans and a sprinkling of dried cranberries or crumbled blue cheese. My wife, Ruth, makes a delicious salad of romaine lettuce, sliced strawberries, and homemade raspberry vinaigrette. It's super easy and very pretty. The salad can be served before the main course to help fill you up, or as one of the side dishes.

Turkey: Prepare a roast turkey for everyone and, for yourself, eat the white breast meat—without the skin, of course. Instead of making a bread-based stuffing, use cooked wild or basmati rice flavored with apples, mushrooms, celery, onions, and herbs.

Vegetables: Choose from the wide array of green-light vegetable dishes. Try roasted, braised, or steamed vegetables in various combinations, with flavorings of lemon, balsamic vinegar, or herbs. Stay away from sauces based in cream, oil, or butter.

Sweet potatoes: If you consider sweet potatoes an essential part of your holiday feast, then go ahead and have them, but instead of adding brown sugar or maple syrup, try ground ginger, light nonhydrogenated margarine, pepper and, instead of cream, hot water or skim milk. But a good baked sweet potato often doesn't need anything at all!

Cranberry sauce: If you make cranberry sauce, replace the sugar in your recipe with Splenda. Ruth always adds some chopped fresh orange and slivered almonds for extra flavor and crunch.

Dessert: Dessert can always be part of a green-light meal! All of my books contain recipes for desserts, and in this volume you can find some delicious selections starting on page 272. A sweet, easy-to-make treat to end your holiday dinner could be a low-fat, no-sugar-added ice cream, fresh berries with sweetened yogurt cheese, poached pears, or a fruit crumble.

Here are some ways e-Clinic participants dealt with the holidays:

"The newest strategy for our Christmas preparation is to focus on establishing new traditions with decorating and doing specific things together instead of the classics from my past that revolved around Christmas treats, such as Toblerone, chocolate oranges, Christmas cake, and so on."

—Bernadette

"This weekend was THE weekend for us for holiday parties. Friday night, Saturday lunch, Saturday night, and Sunday lunch, followed by a concert and dessert reception. . . . I made myself a deal to cope with the events (I had no control over the food available): If I could eat mostly green- and some yellow-light foods, I could have a drink or two. If there were only yellow- or red-light foods available, it was club soda and lime for me."—Karen

"Thanksgiving went fairly well, with boiled new potatoes instead of mashed and smaller portions of white meat only and no seconds."—Ross

"I was pleasantly surprised to get on the scales this morning and find I still weighed the same! One of the things I noticed yesterday was I was not left with that sick, stuffed feeling after the Thanksgiving meal! My biggest challenges were not tasting as I cooked the meal and deciding what to do with the leftovers, which I didn't want to waste. Would I rather they go to my waist? NO! I gave away over half of them. We will have a few sensible meals out of the healthier ones. Some I simply dumped! Yay!"—Diane

"Events such as Thanksgiving, Halloween, and birthdays were always a free ticket to overeat for me—it was almost as though it was expected. This time was different. I still enjoyed the food and celebrations, but when tempted to slide I thought, 'Is it worth having to wait another week or two or more to get to my goal?'"—Kathy

Remember that holidays and joyous celebrations are special not because of the food we serve, but because of the loved ones we're with. The day can easily be special without being red-light.

Week 11 Weight: _____

Week 11 Waist: _____

Week 11 Hips: _____

week 11 diary

WEEK 11 OPTIONAL MEAL PLAN

	BREAKFAST	SNACK	LUNCH
MONDAY	Homey Oatmeal (p. 202) with chopped apple	Apple Bran Muffin (p. 264)	Open-faced chicken sandwich with lettuce, tomato, and onion, and Basic G.I. Salad (p. 215)
TUESDAY	Mini Breakfast Puffs (p. 206)	Fruit yogurt	G.I. Pasta Salad (p. 224)
WEDNESDAY	Homemade Muesli (p. 203) with skim milk and fruit yogurt	Apple Bran Muffin (p. 264)	½ whole wheat pita with canned light tuna, lettuce, tomato, and cucumber, and Basic G.I. Salad (p. 215)
THURSDAY	Homey Oatmeal (p. 202) with blueberries	Small apple and glass of skim milk	Quick and Easy Chicken Noodle Soup (p. 211) and Basic G.I. Salad (p. 215)
FRIDAY	All-Bran Bran Buds (or other high-fiber cereal) with skim milk, peach slices, and sliced almonds	Fruit yogurt	Mixed Bean Salad (p. 222)
SATURDAY	Vegetarian Omelet (p. 209)	½ nutrition bar	Greek Salad (p. 218)
SUNDAY	Oatmeal Buttermilk Pancakes (p. 205) with strawberries	Orange and almonds	Tuscan White Bean Soup (p. 213) and Basic G.I. Salad (p. 215)

Note: You are not required to use these weekly meal plans and shopping lists. Feel free to pick and choose and make up your own green-light meals.

SNACK	DINNER	SNACK
Laughing Cow Light cheese with crispbread	Rigatoni with Mini Meatballs (p. 254) and Caesar Salad (p. 216)	Mixed berries tossed in lime juice with fat-free sour cream
Hummus with carrot and celery sticks	Citrus-Poached Haddock (p. 239), green beans, and new potatoes	Orange and almonds
Babybel Light cheese with crispbread	Chicken Jambalaya (p. 256) and broccoli	Creamy Lemon Square (p. 279) and glass of skim milk
Crunchy Chickpeas (p. 271)	Barley Risotto with Leeks, Lemon, and Peas (p. 236) and Tabbouleh Salad (p. 221)	½ nutrition bar
Laughing Cow Light cheese with crispbread	Thai Red Curry Shrimp Pasta (p. 244)	Mixed berries tossed in lime juice with fat-free sour cream
Hummus with carrot and celery sticks	Zesty Barbecued Chicken (p. 252), Tangy Red and Green Coleslaw (p. 219), and new potatoes	Creamy Lemon Square (p. 279) and glass of fat-free skim milk
Babybel Light cheese with crispbread	Pork Tenderloin with Apple Compote (p. 260), brussels sprouts, carrots, and new potatoes	Piece of Berry Crumble (p. 274)

grocery list for WEEK 11

These ingredients correspond with the recipes in this week's meal plan. Be sure that your basic pantry is well-stocked—refer to the list on pages 46–47.

produce

- ☐ brussels sprouts
- ☐ cabbage, both green and red
- ☐ fresh cilantro
- ☐ eggplant
- ☐ kale
- ☐ leeks
- ☐ iceberg lettuce
- ☐ romaine lettuce
- ☐ fresh mint
- ☐ fresh rosemary
- ☐ fresh sage
- ☐ fresh thyme
- ☐ zucchini

meat, poultry, and fish

- ☐ pork tenderloin
- ☐ skinless, boneless chicken breasts
- ☐ lean ground chicken or turkey
- ☐ haddock fillets
- ☐ large raw shrimp

dairy and deli

- ☐ low-fat cheddar cheese

pastas

- ☐ whole wheat macaroni or small shells
- ☐ whole wheat rigatoni
- ☐ whole wheat rotini or penne
- ☐ whole wheat spaghettini or linguine

miscellaneous

- ☐ dried currants
- ☐ ground cloves
- ☐ ground almonds
- ☐ pecans
- ☐ flax seeds
- ☐ celery seeds
- ☐ bay leaves
- ☐ dried sage
- ☐ kalamata olives
- ☐ Thai red curry paste
- ☐ light tomato sauce with no added sugar
- ☐ frozen apple juice concentrate
- ☐ unsweetened apple juice
- ☐ unsweetened orange juice

week 12:

Exercise

AS THE E-CLINIC PROGRESSED AND THE PARTICIPANTS LOST A considerable amount of weight and found their energy level increasing, many decided to get involved in regular exercise.

"Now that eating is becoming more routine, I want to establish an exercise program. I think this will be important."
—Lynn

"I can almost see the 100s and I am dying to get there! . . . I joined Curves [a fitness club] yesterday."—Beverley

"I am down below what I have been for the past seven years. That is encouraging and I know I will continue the good eating habits I have practiced for the last three months. I also know I am at a place where I need to increase my daily exercise."—Diane

"When my baby was six months old, I tried jogging, but was discouraged when I felt a lot of pain in my shins. This past Thursday, I tried it again and had great success. I have jogged almost every day so far."—Tammy

As we all know, there are many benefits to exercising. Regular exercise will contribute significantly to your health by reducing your risk of heart disease, stroke, diabetes, and osteoporosis; maintaining your muscle mass and tone as you age; and, over the long term, accelerating or maintaining your weight loss. In the United States, the National Weight Control Registry is tracking some 3,000 people who have lost 30 pounds or more and kept it off for six years. One thing these successful dieters have in common is that they are very active and exercise every day. Although exercise is of limited value in helping you achieve your weight-loss target, it becomes a critical factor in helping you maintain your weight and health for the rest of your life. And believe it or not, exercise can be addictive. I tend to become irritable and edgy if I'm not getting my daily exercise fix—or so Ruth tells me. Initially, it can be hard to get out there and hit the sidewalk or gym, but stick with it—the fun will kick in eventually.

I don't want to sound heretical about the value of exercise, but I do find it unfortunate that it has been traditionally put forward as one of the fundamental ways to lose weight. The reality is that you need to exercise an extraordinary amount if you want to lose weight this way. Just take a look at the amount of effort it requires to simply lose 1 pound of fat:

	130-Pound Person	**160-Pound Person**
Walking (brisk; 4 mph)	53 miles/85 km	42 miles/67 km
Running (8 min/mile)	36 miles/58 km	29 miles/46 km
Cycling (12–14 mph)	96 miles/154 km	79 miles/126 km
Sex (moderate effort)	79 times	64 times

This is one reason fitness clubs have such a high turnover rate. People sign up principally because they want to be able to lose weight (which is why fitness club business always booms early in the new year following the excesses of the holiday season). Many, if not most, however, soon find that their exercise regimen is not really shifting those pounds. They become discouraged and drop out. I'm sure some of you have experienced this.

The reality is that in our busy world, walking 53 miles to lose 1 pound of fat, for example, is quite unrealistic for most of us. That is why I suggest that losing weight is 90 percent diet and 10 percent exercise. So focus on changing the way you eat and later, as you approach your target weight, consider introducing an exercise plan as part of your new lifestyle. Exercise is wonderful for helping maintain your weight as well as being essential for your long-term health.

TYPES OF EXERCISE

Before I go any further, I should define exactly what I mean by exercise. There are three basic types, each working in concert with the others.

Aerobic

Aerobic exercise gets your heart and lungs working harder and relies on oxygen, carbohydrates, and fats for its energy. Your progress over time can be measured by increased endurance and decreased fatigue. Aerobic exercises such as walking, jogging, biking, swimming, hiking, and so on will have the most impact on your overall weight and health.

Strength

Strength training, also known as resistance training, will help minimize muscle loss—and in fact will actually help build muscle mass as your body turns to its protein reserves to strengthen and enlarge its musculature. Resistance exercises involve fixed or free weights, elastic bands, or even your own body weight; pushing your hands together as hard as you can is a form of resistance exercise. You don't have to join a gym or work out with massive barbells. A few simple exercises, easily done at home, will work wonders restoring or toning those flabby muscles.

Strength training is particularly important as we move into middle age and beyond because of the steady reduction in muscle mass that accompanies aging. Starting at the age of twenty-five, the body loses 2 percent of its muscle mass each decade, a process that accelerates to 6 to 8 percent as we move into our senior years. Exercising muscles on a regular basis minimizes or reverses the loss. And why is that important? Because the larger your muscles, the more energy (calories) they use. When you're at rest, or even asleep in bed, your muscles are using energy. So keeping or building muscle mass really helps you burn calories and lose weight.

Stretching

Stretching is exactly what it sounds like: the process of "warming up" your body by flexing and moving it. Stretching activities (such as tai chi, yoga, ballet warm-ups, and other gentle movements) will give you the biggest bang for your buck in terms of immediate payoff. Within just a week, you can increase your flexibility by over 100 percent.

Both aerobic exercise and strength training can actually make you less flexible if you don't stretch those muscles, ligaments, and tendons. That's why you see athletes warming up and cooling down with stretching exercises. Always include stretching in your exercise program.

Flexibility is also a significant issue as we age and lose mobility in our joints, tendons, and ligaments. Loss of flexibility reduces our ability to do either aerobic or strength training, both of which depend on healthy joints and tissues. In older people, this loss of flexibility can lead to falls and hip fractures. So although stretching may seem like a "frill," it is central to the whole fitness picture.

Now let's review the various options, each of which ought to incorporate elements of all three types of exercise.

OUTDOOR ACTIVITIES

Walking

This is by far the simplest and, for most people, the easiest exercise program to start and maintain. And you don't need any special clothing or equipment, except a pair of comfortable cushioned shoes. Walking is rarely boring: You can change routes and watch the world go by; you can walk with your spouse, child, or friend for company and mutual support, or go solo and commune with nature and your own thoughts. I prefer to walk on my own in the morning, which is when I do my best thinking.

For adults, an average of thirty minutes of walking a day, seven days a week, should be the target (if you do an hour-long walk one day of the weekend, you can take a day off during the week). We're talking about brisk walking, not speed walking (which can verge on running) or slowly ambling along. Imagine you're late for an appointment, and keep that pace. Your heart and breathing rates should increase, but never to the point where you lack the breath to talk with a partner.

A great idea for working people is to incorporate walking into their daily commute. I found a simple way to get my half hour of walking a day was to get off the bus three stops early on my way to work and walk the extra three stops on my way home. Those three stops were equal to about 1½ miles, so I was walking about 3 miles each day! If you drive to work, try parking your car a few blocks farther away than you normally do and walk the rest of the way to your job. You may even find cheaper parking. Gradually increase the distance and your exercise. Who knows, you may eventually be able to walk to work. Think of the savings in gas and parking fees!

Jogging or Running

This is similar to walking, but you need proper jogging footwear to protect joints from damage. Jogging approximately doubles the number of calories burned in the same period of time as walking: 400 calories for jogging versus 200 for brisk walking over a thirty-minute period. Jogging also increases your heart rate, which is great for heart health. Like all muscles, the heart thrives on exercise, so, in general, the more the better.

To see if it is for you, try jogging for a few intervals while on one of your daily walks—walk five minutes, then jog for one minute. If it feels good, on subsequent walks you can start gradually increasing your jogging time and decreasing your walking time, until you are spending all your time at a nice brisk jogging pace. If jogging suits you, good news! Like walking, this is one of the simplest and most effective methods of exercise—it can be done anywhere and it's inexpensive.

Hiking

Another variation on walking is cross-country hiking—walking outdoors off of paved roads, such as in the mountains or through forests or nature preserves. Because this usually involves different kinds of terrain, especially hills and valleys, you use more calories, about 50 percent more than for brisk walking. (Try hauling 150 to 200 pounds up a hill and you'll get some idea of the extra effort your body has to make.) As with walking and jogging, be sure you have proper hiking footwear, and don't push yourself too hard! You don't want to find yourself on a trail in the middle of the woods with no energy left to get back to your starting point.

Bicycling

Like walking, jogging, and hiking, bicycling is a fun way to burn calories, and it is almost as effective as jogging (for people with low back or knee problems, it can be preferable). Other than the cost of the bike and helmet, it's inexpensive and can be done almost anywhere—with lights and reflectors for night riding, of course. Mountain biking, which is to road biking what hiking is to walking, burns more calories—but also requires more skill and can be more dangerous. Stick to trails and bike paths unless you are an experienced cyclist.

Other Sports

Although most sports are terrific calorie burners, they usually can't be part of a daily routine. Most of them require facilities, equipment, and other people. But they can provide a boost to your regular fitness and exercise program. Such popular sports as tennis, basketball, soccer, softball, and golf (no golf cart, please) are excellent additions to a basic exercise program, and joining a team or league can be a good way to play sports regularly. But though they can be a fun and social supplement to a five- to seven-day-a-week regular exercise schedule, sports are no substitute.

INDOOR ACTIVITIES

Many of you will be muttering by now about how all this would be fine advice if we all lived in southern California, because many of us must contend with either frigid, snowy winters or hot, humid summers, which limit outdoor activities. The alternatives are to either organize a home gym or join a fitness club. The advantage of clubs is that they offer a wide range of sophisticated equipment, with instruction and advice from staff. Clubs are also social, and some people find they need group motivation to work out with enthusiasm. YMCA/YWCAs and some community centers also offer special programs for elderly people, new mothers, and those with special needs; some also provide subsidies for people who can't afford the membership fees. Many centers offer free fitness classes, too.

If a fitness club isn't convenient or if those Lycra-clad young things make you uncomfortable, you can always set up an exercise area at home and invest in some exercise equipment. The best and least expensive piece of equipment is a stationary bike. The latest models work on magnetic resistance rather than on the old friction strap around the flywheel, and this gives a smoother action, with better tension adjustment. Most important, they are quiet, which is crucial if you want to be able to listen to music or watch TV. You can easily pay in the thousands for a bike with all the fancy trimmings, but the $250 to $300 machines will work fine. Just be sure you choose one that has smooth, adjustable tension; then pop in that late-night movie or your favorite soap and get pedaling. Twenty minutes on the bike consumes the same number of calories as thirty minutes of brisk walking, and you'll be amazed how quickly the minutes fly by.

If biking is not for you, try a treadmill. These can be expensive, and beware of the lower-end models that can't take the pounding. Expect to pay about $1,000 and up for something of good quality; you might want to use a day pass to a fitness club to try out their models and note which are most comfortable. Make sure the incline of the track can be raised and lowered for a better workout.

Treadmills and bikes can simulate outdoor walking, jogging, hiking, or biking in the comfort of your own home. I use both of these machines, but have also recently added a cross-country ski machine, which has the advantage of working the upper body as well. Ski machines are generally less expensive than treadmills, but cost more than stationary bikes. They also burn a lot of calories (similar to the amount burned when jogging) because they use the arms and shoulders as well as the legs. Ski machines are almost the perfect all-body workout machine.

There are several other specialized options, such as stair climbers, elliptical walkers, and rowing machines, but they're not for everyone. They are also quite expensive, so try them out first at a fitness club or with a cooperative retailer.

Strength Training

Now it's time to pay attention to rebuilding your muscle mass. Remember that after age forty, you may lose between 4 and 6 pounds of muscle every decade, usually replaced with flab. That's

4 to 6 pounds of calorie-consuming muscle. Muscles burn energy even when idle, and bigger muscles consume more energy than smaller muscles, so they come in handy for losing or maintaining weight.

Resistance-training equipment can range from complex and expensive home gyms to a $10 rubber band. Home gyms, with prices that begin at a couple of hundred dollars and can quickly run up into the thousands, are a popular option. For most people, however, there are cheaper, simpler methods, such as a set of free weights or (my own preference) rubber exercise bands. Dyna-Band and Thera-Band are two popular choices. I like using Thera-Bands, which come in varying thicknesses that offer increasing levels of resistance as you regain and build your muscle strength.

Weights and resistance rubber bands are available at many fitness exercise equipment retailers and surgical supply stores, as well as at online retailers (do an Internet search for "resistance bands"). Try a few resistance exercises, concentrating on the larger muscle groups—your legs, arms, and upper chest. These are the muscles that will give you the biggest bang by burning up the most calories. Resistance exercises are best done every other day, leaving time for your muscles to recuperate, and they should complement your regular exercise regimen, not replace it. Committing to both types of exercise will produce far better results than either one alone.

Pilates

I've recently become a Pilates enthusiast. This very precise system of exercises was originally recommended by my physiotherapist to strengthen my back and prevent my disc problem from recurring. It does a lot more than just that, however. It's a series of floor exercises—no equipment needed—that both strengthen and stretch your muscles, especially the core muscles in your back and around your waist, which are essential for good posture. It's great for any level of fitness and at any age. You can find instructional DVDs at stores and online, and more and more gyms and community centers are now offering Pilates classes.

Yoga and Tai Chi

Yoga comes in different styles, which focus on different elements: balance, breathing, strength, meditation, and so on. If you're new to yoga, the best choice is hatha, which teaches you simple postures that will keep you supple, relax you, and improve your breathing and circulation. But in any form, this ancient practice has much to offer, especially to anyone taking up exercise in middle age.

Tai chi is another Eastern discipline that is gentle, promoting flexibility, balance, and energy. It features a series of flowing postures, done standing, which many people like to practice early in the morning, outdoors. Tai chi keeps the joints and tendons supple and offers a peaceful, revitalizing form of activity that can carry you into old age.

You can read about both yoga and tai chi in books or online, or stop by a community center or yoga studio for more information. Instructional DVDs or videos are also available.

For more suggestions about incorporating physical activity into your daily life, check out the U.S. government's physical activity initiative at http://www.healthierus.gov/exercise.html—there's a wealth of information to be found.

Whether you take up walking, hockey, dance lessons, or nature hikes, make sure it is an activity you enjoy. If you take pleasure from your exercise, you are more likely to do it.

Week 12 Weight: _____

Week 12 Waist: _____

Week 12 Hips: _____

week 12 diary

WEEK 12 OPTIONAL MEAL PLAN

	BREAKFAST	SNACK	LUNCH
MONDAY	Homey Oatmeal (p. 202) with chopped apple	Whole Wheat Fruit Scone (p. 269)	Open-faced lean deli ham sandwich with lettuce, tomato, red pepper, and grainy mustard, and Basic G.I. Salad (p. 215)
TUESDAY	Mini Breakfast Puffs (p. 206)	Fruit yogurt	Waldorf Chicken and Rice Salad (p. 226)
WEDNESDAY	Homemade Muesli (p. 203) with skim milk and fruit yogurt	Whole Wheat Fruit Scone (p. 269)	Cottage cheese with apple and grapes, and Basic G.I. Salad (p. 215)
THURSDAY	Homey Oatmeal (p. 202) with blueberries	Small apple and glass of skim milk	Minestrone (p. 212) and Basic G.I. Salad (p. 215)
FRIDAY	All-Bran Bran Buds (or other high-fiber cereal) with skim milk, peach slices, and sliced almonds	Fruit yogurt	½ whole wheat pita with deli turkey, lettuce, tomato, and cucumber, and Basic G.I. Salad (p. 215)
SATURDAY	Canadian Bacon Omelet (p. 207)	½ nutrition bar	Crab Salad in Tomato Shells (p. 225)
SUNDAY	Cinnamon French Toast (p. 204) with Canadian bacon	Orange and almonds	Ham and Lentil Soup (p. 214) and Basic G.I. Salad (p. 215)

Note: You are not required to use these weekly meal plans and shopping lists. Feel free to pick and choose and make up your own green-light meals.

SNACK	DINNER	SNACK
Laughing Cow Light cheese with crispbread	Salmon Pasta (p. 238)	Mixed berries tossed in lime juice with fat-free sour cream
Hummus with carrot and celery sticks	Pan-Seared Whitefish with Mandarin Salsa (p. 242), broccoli, and basmati rice	Orange and almonds
Babybel Light cheese with crispbread	Chicken Schnitzel (p. 248), green beans, carrots, and new potatoes	Slice of Strawberry Tea Bread (p. 270) and glass of skim milk
Crunchy Chickpeas (p. 271)	Mushroom Gravy Pork Chops (p. 263), asparagus, and basmati rice	½ nutrition bar
Laughing Cow Light cheese with crispbread	Horseradish Burgers (p. 258) and Tabbouleh Salad (p. 221)	Mixed berries tossed in lime juice with fat-free sour cream
Hummus with carrot and celery sticks	Vegetarian Moussaka (p. 232) and basmati rice	Slice of Strawberry Tea Bread (p. 270) and glass of skim milk
Babybel Light cheese with crispbread	Spicy Roast Chicken with Tomatoes and Tarragon (p. 249), green beans, and basmati rice	Slice of One-Bowl Chocolate Cake (p. 276)

grocery list for WEEK 12

These ingredients correspond with the recipes in this week's meal plan. Be sure that your basic pantry is well-stocked—refer to the list on pages 46–47.

produce

- ☐ alfalfa sprouts (optional)
- ☐ asparagus
- ☐ fresh basil
- ☐ fresh cilantro
- ☐ eggplant
- ☐ grapes
- ☐ fresh mint
- ☐ baby spinach
- ☐ fresh tarragon
- ☐ large beefsteak tomatoes
- ☐ cherry or grape tomatoes

meat, poultry, and fish

- ☐ extra-lean ground beef
- ☐ boneless pork loin chops
- ☐ Canadian bacon
- ☐ skinless, boneless chicken breasts
- ☐ canned crab
- ☐ salmon fillet
- ☐ whitefish fillets

dairy and deli

- ☐ low-fat, low-sugar buttermilk salad dressing
- ☐ light herb and garlic cream cheese
- ☐ lean deli ham
- ☐ lean deli turkey

pastas

- ☐ whole wheat macaroni or small shells

miscellaneous

- ☐ dried apricots
- ☐ sun-dried tomatoes
- ☐ dried basil
- ☐ Italian herb seasoning
- ☐ prepared horseradish
- ☐ pecans
- ☐ walnuts
- ☐ unsweetened apple juice
- ☐ unsweetened orange juice
- ☐ whole wheat bread crumbs
- ☐ whole wheat hamburger buns

week 13:

When Weight Loss Causes Anxiety

ON THIS, THE FINAL WEEK OF YOUR THREE-MONTH JOURNEY on the G.I. Diet, I would like to talk about the influence of social factors on the weight-loss experience. At the beginning of the e-Clinic, many participants told me that they didn't want their family, friends, and coworkers to know they were trying to lose weight.

> *"I have not told any coworkers and only two close friends about being on the program because of the fear of the 'I told you so,' 'I knew you'd never stick to it,' and 'You're on another diet?' responses I have heard all my life from my mother and others. . . . Social situations are still uncomfortable for me and I am very self-conscious about how I look."*—Kathy

"In group situations (especially with family), if I'm not eating what other people are eating, then people are going to talk. They're going to start asking me if I'm on a diet, and I don't want to admit that I am, because my low self-esteem says that I'm not going to be able to do it, and then everyone will talk about what a failure I am."—Lynette

"I often feel self-conscious because of my size and appearance, so what better way to bury these bad feelings than with my old friend and comfort blanket: lots of food? Also, I avoid calling attention to myself by reverting to old eating patterns so no one asks why I'm not overeating as usual, in other words acting normal to avoid scrutiny."—Ross

The anxiety that the e-Clinic participants felt at the beginning often doesn't disappear as the diet begins to take effect; instead, it takes a different form. Anxiety about being caught failing and feeling humiliated can be heightened when people start noticing your weight loss and ask questions like, "Have you lost some weight?" or "What diet are you trying now?" You might start to feel like you're being watched and like people are wondering how long it will be before you give up. This is especially true if you have been a yo-yo dieter.

The best defense in this case is to have a set of responses ready for their comments:

- "Thank you for noticing."
- "Thanks. I'm going to need your support as I do this."
- "I know you want me to succeed so I can improve my health. Let me tell you how you can help."
- "Thanks, I found a new way of eating and it really seems to be working."

Sadly, family members can sometimes be the most discouraging. Here is an example from Pat:

> *"When my sister met me to drive me home, she commented on how she could tell that I had lost a significant amount of weight. That made me feel great. I said, 'Oh that reminds me that I have some dress pants that are getting too big.' Her response was, 'Oh just put them in a box—you never know when you will need them again.' Horrified, I said I would never need them again. How is that for a little encouragement and discouragement all at the same time?"*

If you become the target of dispiriting comments like those Pat heard, or ones like "So what's the magic diet this time around?" or "How long will the weight be off this time?" try squelching them with kindness. Say something like, "Jim, I'm sure you want me to succeed, so saying something supportive would be much more helpful." Then smile—you'll feel better for taking the high road.

Whether others are supportive or skeptical, it's quite possible that you yourself will be experiencing some anxiety about changing your body. Strange though it may seem when our greatest wish is often to be slim and trim, deep down many people worry that they won't recognize their new self and that they won't be the same person.

Does your personality change when you lose weight? Certainly you may feel healthier, have more energy, sleep better, worry less, and feel less depressed, but none of this has anything to do with your personality, which is formed early on and makes you one of a kind, different from everyone else. Your personality is essentially who you are, and it's not going to change when you lose weight. If you have a wicked sense of humor, it's not going to disappear when you lose a hundred pounds. If you are shy, losing weight isn't going to turn you into a party animal. You may feel more comfortable in social situations, but you will still be you. Some of the defensive behaviors you developed to survive being large in the world may disappear with the pounds, but the fundamental you will remain.

Excess weight is often subconsciously used to hide and protect the body. Ironically, being large can make people "invisible"—that is, unnoticed or ignored. It can be a way to desexualize the body, in that men and women can deemphasize their sexual and gender-specific physical qualities. For example, women with histories of sexual abuse have been known to become heavy—unconsciously or consciously—as a means of protection, inspired by the notion that men will not be attracted to a large, asexual body. (This involves very complex psychological issues that are beyond the scope of this book.)

For all who have been large, regardless of their sex, losing excess weight can give the body a defined shape, making women look more traditionally feminine and men more traditionally masculine. They may suddenly be seen and noticed, and considered physically attractive or "sexy," which may be anxiety-producing.

But the reality is that it's a whole lot easier living in this society when your body is not overweight. Slender people tend to be treated better than overweight people, and research findings show that slender people are regarded as being brighter, richer, and happier than those who are overweight and also that people who are attractive advance more quickly in the workplace.

Once you've lost a significant amount of weight and bought yourself a new wardrobe, you might find yourself receiving more attention, both at work and socially. Be prepared. You might want to start practicing how you will behave in these new situations. A number of e-Clinic participants wrote me about some of their experiences as the weight came off:

"When people comment on my changing appearance . . . it is sometimes difficult to suppress that inner voice that tends to 'overthink' things, and this leads to misinterpretation of a simple compliment. There are undeniable emotionally laden aspects to this process that lead to veering off the path, so to speak."—Bernadette

"So many people in my office have now bought your book (I bet at least nine people) and come to me regularly for help and guidance. It is so funny. They are all amazed at the physical transition. I wore low-waisted jeans last week and felt like a monkey in a zoo. People were coming by to look at me because someone else would say, 'Have you seen Bev today? She looks great.' I found it a little embarrassing. I kept apologizing and saying, 'Well, I still have a lot to lose.' My girlfriend told me to accept it and just say thanks, because I've worked hard and it shows. (She is a big support.)" —Beverley

Become used to the positive attention by doing some role-playing with a close friend. Have him or her comment on how good you look, pay you compliments, ask you out—whatever scenario you might find difficult—and practice your responses. If someone comments on how good you look or likes your new outfit, practice looking that person straight in the eye and saying thank you—no qualifying statements, please!

As you start to become familiar with, and make friends with, your new body, remember that it is okay to retain some insecurities. Virtually all people are dissatisfied with their bodies—even those whose bodies seem perfect. Slim, beautiful people are all too often filled with self-doubt and on the lookout for that new lotion or potion that will improve their appearance. Where would the beauty industry be without all our anxieties? So don't think you're the only one worrying while everyone else feels secure about themselves. We all wish we could be better somehow. Just enjoy your lighter body, and remember that the goal is not perfection, but rather a more comfortable and healthy self.

Well, dear reader, by now you have completed a three-month journey on the G.I. Diet. You may have reached your target weight, or you may still have some way to go. In the next chapter, we'll discuss how to transition your green-light eating through week 14 and beyond.

Week 13 Weight: _____

Week 13 Waist: _____

Week 13 Hips: _____

week 13 diary

_____

_____

_____

_____

_____

_____

_____

_____

_____

_____

_____

_____

WEEK 13 OPTIONAL MEAL PLAN

	BREAKFAST	SNACK	LUNCH
MONDAY	Homey Oatmeal (p. 202) with chopped apple	Cranberry Cinnamon Bran Muffin (p. 266)	Open-faced chicken sandwich with lettuce, tomato, and onion, and Basic G.I. Salad (p. 215)
TUESDAY	Mini Breakfast Puffs (p. 206)	Fruit yogurt	G.I. Pasta Salad (p. 224)
WEDNESDAY	Homemade Muesli (p. 203) with skim milk and fruit yogurt	Cranberry Cinnamon Bran Muffin (p. 266)	½ whole wheat pita with canned light tuna, lettuce, tomato, and cucumber, and Basic G.I. Salad (p. 215)
THURSDAY	Homey Oatmeal (p. 202) with blueberries	Small apple and glass of skim milk	Quick and Easy Chicken Noodle Soup (p. 211) and Basic G.I. Salad (p. 215)
FRIDAY	All-Bran Bran Buds (or other high-fiber cereal) with skim milk, peach slices, and sliced almonds	Fruit yogurt	Mixed Bean Salad (p. 222)
SATURDAY	Western Omelet (p. 210)	½ nutrition bar	Greek Salad (p. 218)
SUNDAY	Oatmeal Buttermilk Pancakes (p. 205) with strawberries	Orange and almonds	Tuscan White Bean Soup (p. 213) and Basic G.I. Salad (p. 215)

Note: You are not required to use these weekly meal plans and shopping lists. Feel free to pick and choose and make up your own green-light meals.

SNACK	DINNER	SNACK
Laughing Cow Light cheese with crispbread	Easy-Bake Lasagna (p. 228) and Caesar Salad (p. 216)	Mixed berries tossed in lime juice with fat-free sour cream
Hummus with carrot and celery sticks	G.I. Fish Fillet (p. 237), asparagus, carrots, and new potatoes	Orange and almonds
Babybel Light cheese with crispbread	Chicken Curry (p. 247) and Raita Salad (p. 220)	Apple Pie Cookie (p. 278) and glass of skim milk
Crunchy Chickpeas (p. 271)	Vegetable Crumble (p. 230) and Tabbouleh Salad (p. 221)	½ nutrition bar
Laughing Cow Light cheese with crispbread	Fried Rice with Chicken (p. 246)	Mixed berries tossed in lime juice with fat-free sour cream
Hummus with carrot and celery sticks	Beef and Eggplant Chili (p. 257) and Basic G.I. Salad (p. 215)	Apple Pie Cookie (p. 278) and glass of skim milk
Babybel Light cheese with crispbread	Pork Medallions Dijon (p. 261), green beans, carrots, and new potatoes	Piece of Plum Crumble (p. 275)

grocery list for WEEK 13

These ingredients correspond with the recipes in this week's meal plan. Be sure that your basic pantry is well-stocked—refer to the list on pages 46–47.

produce

- ☐ asparagus
- ☐ bean sprouts
- ☐ eggplant
- ☐ kale
- ☐ leeks
- ☐ iceberg lettuce
- ☐ romaine lettuce
- ☐ fresh mint
- ☐ prune plums
- ☐ sweet potatoes
- ☐ fresh sage
- ☐ baby spinach
- ☐ fresh tarragon
- ☐ fresh thyme
- ☐ firm tofu
- ☐ zucchini

meat, poultry, and fish

- ☐ extra-lean ground beef
- ☐ pork tenderloins
- ☐ Canadian bacon
- ☐ skinless, boneless chicken breasts
- ☐ fish fillets, such as salmon or trout

dairy and deli

- ☐ low-fat cheddar cheese
- ☐ part-skim mozzarella cheese

pastas

- ☐ whole wheat lasagna
- ☐ whole wheat rotini or penne

miscellaneous

- ☐ dried cranberries
- ☐ raisins
- ☐ kalamata olives
- ☐ flax seeds
- ☐ sesame seeds
- ☐ mixed nuts
- ☐ ground cardamom
- ☐ curry powder
- ☐ light tomato sauce with no added sugar
- ☐ low-fat tomato pasta sauce

beyond week 13:

Phase II

NOW THAT YOU'RE DONE WITH THE THIRTEEN WEEKS OF THE Clinic, you probably find yourself in one of two situations: Either you've made it to your goal weight, or you've still got a bit more to go.

If you still have extra pounds to shed, I advise you to continue using the Phase I eating plan, as you have for the past three months, and to continue taking weekly measurements and weighing yourself weekly. You can turn back to the shopping lists and menus in the previous weeks for guidance and instruction (for some variety in the menus, you can also check out my other books, *The G.I. Diet* and *Living the G.I. Diet*, both of which have a wealth of recipes). Once you've made it to your goal weight, come back to this chapter to learn about Phase II: maintenance.

If you're one of those who has made it to your target weight in thirteen weeks, congratulations! You've hit your goal, you're wearing clothes you thought you'd never get into again, and you're finally on good terms with your full-length mirror. I hope you are relishing the new you and making the most of your increased energy. Now you can ease up a bit on limiting portion and serving sizes, and start adding some yellow-light foods to your diet—in short, you can graduate from Phase I of the G.I. Diet and move into Phase II. The idea here is maintenance, so it's important that you get comfortable with your G.I. program: This is how you're going to eat for the rest of your life.

PHASE II SERVING SIZES: MODERATION IS KEY

Phase II, I must warn you, is a bit of a danger zone. This is the stage of any diet when things can go off the rails. Some people think that when they reach their weight-loss goal, they can just drop the strict rules of the diet and go back to their old eating habits. And, frankly, when I take a close look at what many of these other diets expect you to live on, I can understand why people can't stick to them for long.

The reality is that, with some modifications, the G.I. program is your diet for life. But this shouldn't be a hardship, because the G.I. Diet was designed to give you a huge range of healthy choices, so you won't feel hungry, bored, or unsatisfied. By now you know how to navigate your green-light way through the supermarket, select green-light foods in restaurants, and cook the green-light way. You are likely not even tempted to revert to your old ways. If you should fall prey to a double cheeseburger (that good old $10 cure), you will be dismayed at how heavy, sluggish, and ungratified you feel afterward. You will be too attached to your new feeling of lightness and level of energy to abandon them.

Before we look at some of the new options open to you in Phase II, a word of caution: Your body can now function on less food than it did before you started. Why? Because you're lighter now, so your body requires fewer calories. Also, your metabolism has become more efficient, and your body has learned to do more with fewer calories. Keeping these two developments in mind, although it's okay to add a few more calories in Phase II, don't go berserk. Don't make any significant changes in your serving sizes, and remember to make yellow-light foods the exception rather than the rule. This way, you will keep the balance between the calories you're consuming and the calories you're expending—and that is the secret to maintaining your new weight.

As you modestly increase portions of foods that you particularly enjoy and include some yellow-light items as a treat, keep monitoring your weight weekly, and adjust your servings up or down until your weight stays stable. This may take a few weeks of experimentation, but when you've reached the magic balance and can stay there comfortably, that's the formula for the rest of your days.

The best news for most of us in Phase II is the reintroduction of alcohol and chocolate. While both were strictly off-limits in both the Preliminary Phase and Phase I because of their high calorie content and tendency to spike blood sugar levels, in Phase II, it's time to reintroduce those little pleasures.

Alcohol

Medical research indicates that red wine, which is rich in flavonoids, can help reduce your risk of heart disease and stroke. So in Phase II, a glass of red wine is allowed with dinner. Just because one glass is beneficial, however, doesn't mean that having two or three is even better for you. The negative side effects of immoderate drinking undo any health benefits of that glass-a-day, and alcohol contains calories. One glass of wine (5 ounces maximum) provides the optimum benefit.

Apart from red wine, keep your consumption of alcohol to a minimum. I realize that this can be difficult, because drinking is so often a part of social occasions and celebrations. An occasional lapse won't do a lot of harm, but it's easy to get carried away. There are various strategies to combat the social pressure to drink: You can graciously accept that glass of wine or cocktail, raise it in a toast, take a sip, and then discreetly leave it on the nearest buffet table. Faced with a tray of vodka martinis and glasses of red wine, stick with the wine, which lasts longer. Ruth drinks spritzers (wine mixed with soda water) on special occasions. And if you add lots of ice to your spritzer, you can reduce the alcohol even further while still joining in the party spirit. Whatever strategy you choose, always try to eat some food with your drink, even if it has to be a forbidden piece of cheese. The fat will slow the absorption of the alcohol and minimize its impact. (Of course, better to gravitate to the vegetable tray, but an emergency canapé won't be the ruin of you.)

Chocolate

For many of us, living without chocolate is not living. The good news is that in Phase II, some chocolate—the right sort of chocolate in the right amount—is acceptable. You may have heard that chocolate, like red wine, contains natural elements that help keep the arteries clear—but that's probably not your main motive for eating it. Chocolate combines fat, sugar, and cocoa, all three of which please the palate. But most chocolate contains too much saturated fat and sugar, which keeps it deep in the red-light zone. Chocolate with a high cocoa content (dark or bittersweet chocoloate, or chocolate advertised as containing 70 percent or more cocoa) delivers more chocolate intensity per ounce, which means that even a square or two is satisfying and can give chocoholics the fix they need.

Here are some other suggestions for ways you can relax your Phase I restrictions for everyday eating in Phase II:

Breakfast

- Increase cereal serving size from ½ to ⅔ of a cup.
- Add a slice of 100% whole-grain toast and a pat of margarine.
- Double the amount of sliced almonds on your cereal.
- Enjoy an extra slice of Canadian bacon.
- Have a glass of unsweetened juice now and then.
- Add one of the yellow-light fruits—a banana or apricot—to your cereal.
- Go caffeinated in the coffee department, if you like, but still try to keep it to one cup a day.

Lunch

I suggest you continue to eat lunch as you did in Phase I, because this is the one meal that already contained some compromises in the weight-loss portion of the program.

Dinner

- Add another boiled new potato to your plate.
- Increase the pasta serving from ¾ cup to 1 cup.
- As a special treat, occasionally have a 6-ounce steak instead of a 4-ounce one.
- Eat a few more olives and nuts—but only a few, as these are calorie heavyweights!
- Try a cob of sweet corn with a dab of nonhydrogenated margarine.
- Have a glass of red wine with dinner.
- Add another slice of high-fiber bread or crispbread.
- Enjoy a yellow-light cut of lamb or pork.

Snacks

- Have a maximum of 2 cups of air-popped popcorn.
- Increase your serving size of nuts to ten or twelve.
- Enjoy a square or two of 70 percent dark chocolate.
- Have a banana.
- Indulge in a scoop of low-fat ice cream or frozen yogurt.
- Eat a whole nutrition bar rather than half a bar.

Of course, Phase II is not, and shouldn't be, a straitjacket. If you live 90 percent within the guidelines of the diet, you are doing well. The idea that certain foods are completely and forever forbidden would sooner or later drive you back into their clutches. With the G.I. Diet, you are in control of what you eat, and that includes (with discipline, moderation, and common sense) almost everything.

WHERE TO GO FROM HERE

Whether you have reached your weight-loss target by now and are ready to start Phase II of the G.I. Diet, or still have some way to go, I would like to offer you what the original participants were offered at the end of the first thirteen weeks of the e-Clinic: a nine-month extension of the program, which includes a monthly e-letter. These monthly e-letters will cover issues such as:

- How to stay the course
- Anxiety and fear of failure
- Maintaining motivation
- Dealing with temptation
- Five essentials to permanent weight loss

Whether they wished to maintain their weight, or still had more weight to lose, the original e-Clinic members found this extension of the basic thirteen-week program extremely valuable. If you'd like to receive these nine monthly e-letters and record your progress on an optional personal website diary, all you have to do is register at www.gidietclinic.com (please note that there is a fee).

An exclusive website will support you during these nine months through a special members' question-and-answer forum, where I will respond to major issues raised in participants' diaries. In addition, you will receive access to a special Green Light Forum where you can share your own experiences with other readers.

Once you register at www.gidietclinic.com, you will receive the first e-letter immediately, as well as access to your personal diary should you wish to track your results. All of your personal information will be kept strictly confidential, and any use of your questions or comments on the website will refer to your first name only.

The e-Clinic is a great opportunity to continue your positive experience with the G.I. Diet. For those of you who do not intend to continue with the nine-month extension, I would be most grateful if you would forward me your weekly results from the thirteen weeks in this book. If this is too much trouble, then just send me your starting measurements and your Week 13 measurements. Simply go to www.gidietclinic.com and click on the link to submit your results through a simple form. Any comments you might have would also be greatly appreciated.

TO SUM UP

- In Phase II, use moderation and common sense in adjusting portions and servings.
- Don't view Phase II as a straitjacket. Occasional lapses are fine.

Part Three

The Recipes

BREAKFAST

Homey Oatmeal

This hot breakfast is guaranteed to keep you feeling satisfied all morning. You can vary the flavor by topping it with fresh fruit, such as berries or chopped apple.

2 cups skim milk
¾ teaspoon ground cinnamon
½ teaspoon salt
1⅓ cups old-fashioned rolled oats
¼ cup wheat germ
¼ cup chopped almonds
3 tablespoons Splenda

Place the milk, cinnamon, salt, and 1½ cups of water in a large pot and bring to a boil. Stir in the oats and wheat germ and let return to a boil. Reduce the heat to low and cook, stirring, until thickened, about 8 minutes. Stir in the almonds and Splenda.

Serves 4

Homemade Muesli

This cereal makes a delicious and healthy start to the day. Be sure to prepare it the night before so that it's ready to enjoy in the morning. Combine one-third cup of the muesli with one-third cup of skim milk or water, cover it, and refrigerate overnight. Then, in the morning, combine the mixture with a container (6 ounces) of nonfat, sugar-free fruit yogurt and enjoy it cold, or pop it in the microwave for a hot breakfast.

2 cups old-fashioned rolled oats
¾ cup oat bran
¾ cup sliced almonds
½ cup shelled unsalted sunflower seeds
2 tablespoons wheat germ
¼ teaspoon ground cinnamon

Combine the oats, oat bran, almonds, sunflower seeds, wheat germ, and cinnamon in a large resealable plastic bag. Using a rolling pin, crush the mixture into coarse crumbs. Shake the bag to mix the muesli well.

Makes 3 cups

Cinnamon French Toast

Serve this family favorite with slices of lean ham or Canadian bacon and extra strawberries for a complete breakfast.

¾ cup liquid egg
½ cup skim milk
1 tablespoon Splenda
1 teaspoon vanilla
½ teaspoon ground cinnamon
Pinch of salt
4 slices stone-ground whole wheat bread
1 teaspoon canola oil
2 cups sliced strawberries
½ cup nonfat sugar-free fruit-flavored yogurt

1. Whisk the liquid egg, milk, Splenda, vanilla, cinnamon, and salt together in a shallow dish. Dip each slice of bread into the egg mixture, making sure to coat both sides.

2. Meanwhile, brush the oil on a nonstick griddle or large nonstick frying pan and heat over medium-high heat. Cook the French toast, turning once, until golden brown on both sides, about 4 minutes. Serve it with the strawberries and yogurt.

Serves 2

Oatmeal Buttermilk Pancakes

Make pancake breakfasts a weekend tradition. Serve them with fresh fruit or applesauce.

¾ cup old-fashioned rolled oats
2 cups buttermilk
1 cup whole wheat flour
¼ cup ground flaxseed
1 tablespoon Splenda
1 teaspoon ground cinnamon
1 teaspoon baking soda
1 teaspoon baking powder
¼ teaspoon salt
½ cup liquid egg
2 tablespoons canola oil
1 teaspoon vanilla

1. Place the oats and the buttermilk in a bowl and let soak for 20 minutes.

2. Combine the whole wheat flour, flaxseed, Splenda, cinnamon, baking soda, baking powder, and salt in a bowl.

3. Place the liquid egg, oil, and vanilla in another bowl and whisk them together. Stir in the soaked oats and buttermilk. Pour the oat mixture over the flour mixture and stir until just mixed.

4. Heat a nonstick griddle or large nonstick frying pan over medium heat. Ladle about ¼ cup of batter onto the griddle for each pancake. Cook until bubbles appear on the top, about 2 minutes.

5. Flip the pancakes and cook them until golden, about 2 minutes longer. Transfer the pancakes to a plate and cover to keep warm. Repeat with the remaining batter.

Makes 16 pancakes; serves 4 to 6

Mini Breakfast Puffs

Ideal for rushed mornings, these muffin-sized puffs are packed with nutrition.

1 teaspoon canola oil
¼ cup diced onion
1 red bell pepper, diced
1 cup chopped broccoli
1½ teaspoons fresh thyme
¼ teaspoon salt
¼ teaspoon freshly ground pepper
¾ cup crumbled light feta cheese
1½ cups liquid egg
1 cup skim milk
¼ cup wheat bran
¼ cup whole wheat flour

1. Preheat the oven to 400°F. Grease a 12-cup muffin tin.

2. Heat the oil in a nonstick frying pan over medium heat. Cook the onion and bell pepper until softened, about 5 minutes. Add the broccoli, thyme, salt, and ground pepper; cover, and let steam until the broccoli is crisp-tender and bright green, about 3 minutes. Divide the vegetable mixture among the muffin cups.

3. Sprinkle some of the feta cheese over the vegetable mixture in each muffin cup, dividing it evenly.

4. Place the liquid egg, milk, wheat bran, and whole wheat flour in a bowl and whisk them together. Spoon the egg mixture evenly over the vegetable mixture, dividing it equally among the muffin cups. Bake the puffs until golden, set, and puffed, about 20 minutes. Let cool slightly before serving.

Makes 12 puffs; serves 6 to 8

Canadian Bacon Omelet

The smoky flavor of Canadian bacon makes this omelet a hit. Serve it with fresh fruit and yogurt for a hearty breakfast.

1 teaspoon canola oil
½ cup liquid egg
1 tablespoon chopped fresh basil
1 tablespoon grated Parmesan cheese
Pinch of freshly ground pepper
2 slices Canadian bacon or lean ham, chopped
¼ red or green bell pepper, chopped

1. Heat the oil in a small nonstick frying pan over medium-high heat. Place the liquid egg, basil, Parmesan cheese, and ground pepper in a bowl and, using a fork, stir them together. Pour the egg mixture into the frying pan and cook until almost set, about 5 minutes, lifting the edges to allow the uncooked egg to run underneath.

2. Sprinkle the Canadian bacon and red or green bell pepper over half of the omelet. Using a spatula, fold over the other half and cook for 1 minute.

Serves 1

Italian Omelet

Omelets are easy to make, and you can vary them by adding any number of fresh vegetables, a little cheese, and/or some meat.

1 teaspoon canola oil
½ cup sliced mushrooms
½ cup liquid egg
½ cup tomato puree
1 tablespoon chopped fresh basil or oregano
1 ounce part-skim mozzarella cheese, shredded
Pinch of freshly ground pepper

1. Heat the oil in a small nonstick frying pan over medium-high heat. Add the mushrooms and cook until tender, about 5 minutes. Transfer the mushrooms to a plate and cover to keep warm.

2. Place the liquid egg, tomato puree, basil, mozzarella cheese, and pepper in a bowl and, using a fork, stir them together. Pour the egg mixture into the frying pan and cook until almost set, about 5 minutes, lifting the edges to allow the uncooked egg to run underneath.

3. Sprinkle the cooked mushrooms over half of the omelet. Using a spatula, fold over the other half and cook for 1 minute.

Serves 1

Vegetarian Omelet

This omelet is open to many variations, and you can also make it with leftover vegetables. Or try adding a small amount of cubed firm tofu when you sauté the vegetables.

1 teaspoon canola oil
1 cup broccoli florets
½ cup sliced mushrooms
½ cup chopped red and green bell pepper
½ cup liquid egg
1 ounce low-fat cheddar cheese, shredded
Pinch of freshly ground pepper

1. Heat the oil in a small nonstick frying pan over medium-high heat. Add the broccoli, mushrooms, and red and green pepper and cook until tender, about 5 minutes. Transfer the vegetables to a plate and cover to keep warm.

2. Place the liquid egg, cheddar cheese, and ground pepper in a bowl and, using a fork, stir them together. Pour the egg mixture into the frying pan and cook until almost set, about 5 minutes, lifting the edges to allow the uncooked egg to run underneath.

3. Sprinkle the cooked vegetables over half of the omelet. Using a spatula, fold over the other half and cook for 1 minute.

Serves 1

Western Omelet

Pair this omelet with a salad and it makes a great weekend brunch.

1 teaspoon canola oil
1 cup chopped red and green bell pepper
1 small onion, chopped
½ cup liquid egg
2 slices Canadian bacon, lean deli ham, or turkey breast, chopped
Pinch of red pepper flakes or cayenne pepper

1. Heat the oil in a small nonstick frying pan over medium-high heat. Add the red and green bell pepper and onion and cook until tender, about 5 minutes. Transfer the vegetables to a plate and cover to keep warm.

2. Place the liquid egg, Canadian bacon, and red pepper flakes in a bowl and, using a fork, stir them together. Pour the egg mixture into the frying pan and cook until almost set, about 5 minutes, lifting the edges to allow the uncooked egg to run underneath.

3. Sprinkle the cooked vegetables over half of the omelet. Using a spatula, fold over the other half and cook for 1 minute.

Serves 1

SOUPS

Quick and Easy Chicken Noodle Soup

Why buy canned chicken soup when you can make this simple homemade version?

2 teaspoons extra-virgin olive oil
2 carrots, chopped
2 ribs celery, chopped
3 cloves garlic, chopped
1 onion, chopped
1 tablespoon chopped fresh thyme
6 cups low-fat, low-sodium chicken broth
3 skinless, boneless half chicken breasts (4 ounces each), diced
1 cup frozen peas
¾ cup small pasta, such as ditali or tubetti
¼ cup chopped fresh flat-leaf parsley
¼ teaspoon salt
¼ teaspoon freshly ground pepper

1. Heat the oil in a large soup pot over medium-high heat. Add the carrots, celery, garlic, onion, and thyme and cook until the vegetables are slightly softened, about 10 minutes.

2. Pour in the chicken broth and bring to a boil. Reduce the heat to a simmer and add the chicken, peas, and pasta. Let simmer until the chicken is no longer pink inside and the pasta is al dente, about 15 minutes. Stir in the parsley, salt, and pepper.

Serves 6

Minestrone

This soup is one of my favorites because it contains both pasta and spinach. Serve it with a sprinkling of grated Parmesan cheese for extra flavor and with a few more red pepper flakes to get your blood pumping.

2 teaspoons canola oil
3 slices Canadian bacon, chopped
1 onion, chopped
4 cloves garlic, minced
2 carrots, chopped
1 rib celery, chopped
1 tablespoon dried oregano
½ teaspoon red pepper flakes
¼ teaspoon salt
¼ teaspoon freshly ground pepper
1 can (28 ounces) plum tomatoes
6 cups low-fat, low-sodium chicken broth
1 package (11 ounces) baby spinach
1 can (15½ ounces) red kidney beans, rinsed and drained
1 can (15½ ounces) chickpeas (garbanzo beans), rinsed and drained
¾ cup ditali or tubetti pasta
⅓ cup chopped fresh flat-leaf parsley
2 tablespoons chopped fresh basil (optional)

1. Heat the oil in a large soup pot over medium-high heat and cook the Canadian bacon for 2 minutes. Reduce the heat to medium and add the onion, garlic, carrots, celery, oregano, red pepper flakes, salt, and ground pepper. Cook until the vegetables are softened and lightly browned, about 10 minutes.

2. Add the tomatoes and, using a potato masher, crush them in the pot. Pour in the chicken broth, then bring to a boil. Reduce the heat to a simmer and add the spinach, kidney beans, chickpeas, and pasta. Let simmer until the pasta is tender, about 20 minutes. Stir in the parsley and basil, if using.

Serves 6

Tuscan White Bean Soup

Serve this soup in deep Italian ceramic soup bowls and dream you're in Tuscany.

1 tablespoon extra-virgin olive oil
1 onion, chopped
4 cloves garlic, minced
1 carrot, chopped
1 rib celery, chopped
4 fresh sage leaves, or ½ teaspoon dried sage
6 cups low-fat, low-sodium vegetable or chicken broth
2 cans (15½ ounces each) cannellini or white kidney beans, rinsed and drained
4 cups shredded kale
Pinch of salt
Pinch of freshly ground pepper

1. Heat the oil in a large soup pot over medium heat. Add the onion, garlic, carrot, celery, and sage and cook until softened, about 5 minutes.

2. Add the broth, beans, kale, salt, and pepper, and cook, stirring occasionally, until the kale is tender, about 20 minutes.

Serves 4

Ham and Lentil Soup

Canned lentils make this soup quick and easy to prepare, so keep some on hand. If you want to make the soup even more green-light, use dried lentils instead (see the instructions in the Variation below).

1 tablespoon canola oil
1 onion, chopped
½ cup diced celery
2 cloves garlic, minced
6 cups low-fat, low-sodium chicken broth
2 cans (15 ounces each) lentils, drained and rinsed
6 ounces black forest ham, diced
1 red bell pepper, diced
2 tomatoes, seeded and diced
2 tablespoons chopped fresh flat-leaf parsley

Heat the oil in a large soup pot over medium heat. Add the onion, celery, and garlic and cook until softened, about 5 minutes. Add the chicken broth, lentils, ham, and bell pepper and bring to a boil. Reduce the heat and add the tomatoes. Cover and let simmer for 20 minutes. Stir in the parsley.

Serves 4

Variation: Use 1 cup of dried green or brown lentils. Add the lentils with the chicken broth, cover the pot, and continue with the recipe, letting the soup simmer until the lentils are tender, about 30 minutes.

SALADS

Basic G.I. Salad

Use this recipe as a guide for making a range of salads with the vegetables of your choice and the different vinegars in the dressing. For a pretty variation of the salad, instead of the vegetables mix soft salad leaves with sliced strawberries, sliced pears, sliced almonds, and a balsamic dressing.

For the salad

1½ cups torn or coarsely chopped greens: arugula, baby spinach, or watercress; Boston, iceberg, leaf, or romaine lettuce; or mesclun
1 small carrot, grated
½ red, yellow, or green bell pepper, diced
1 plum tomato, cut into wedges
½ cup sliced cucumber
¼ cup chopped red onion (optional)

For the Basic G.I. Vinaigrette

1 tablespoon vinegar, such as balsamic, cider, red wine, rice, or white wine vinegar, or 1 tablespoon lemon juice
1 teaspoon extra-virgin olive oil or canola oil
½ teaspoon Dijon mustard
1 clove garlic (optional), peeled and crushed
Pinch of salt
Pinch of freshly ground pepper
Pinch of finely chopped fresh herb of choice, such as basil, marjoram, mint, oregano, or thyme

1. Make the salad: Place the lettuce, carrot, bell pepper, tomato, cucumber, and onion, if using, in a large bowl and toss them together.

2. Make the Basic G.I. Vinaigrette: Place the vinegar, oil, mustard, garlic, if using, salt, ground pepper, and herb in a small bowl and whisk them together.

3. Pour the vinaigrette over the greens and toss to coat.

Serves 1

Variations: To make a meal out of this salad, add some protein with 4 ounces of canned tuna, cooked salmon, tofu, kidney beans, chickpeas, or cooked chicken or another lean meat.

Make Ahead: Both the salad and the dressing can be prepared ahead and refrigerated separately, covered, for about 2 days.

Caesar Salad

We all need a Caesar salad in our recipe repertoire. No one will guess that tahini is the secret ingredient that makes this green-light version every bit as creamy as chef Caesar Cardini's original.

For the salad

3 slices whole-grain bread
2 teaspoons extra-virgin olive oil
Pinch of salt
Pinch of freshly ground pepper
1 large head romaine lettuce

For the dressing

3 cloves garlic, minced
3 anchovy fillets, finely minced
2 tablespoons tahini
1 teaspoon Dijon mustard
½ teaspoon Worcestershire sauce
½ teaspoon salt
½ teaspoon freshly ground pepper
3 tablespoons fresh lemon juice
2 tablespoons warm water
1½ tablespoons extra-virgin olive oil

1. Preheat the oven to 350°F.

2. Make the salad: Cut the bread into ½-inch pieces and place them in a bowl. Add the 2 teaspoons of olive oil, the pinch of salt, and the pinch of pepper and toss to coat well. Arrange the bread in a single layer on a rimmed baking sheet. Bake the bread until golden and crisp, about 20 minutes. Let cool.

3. Rinse the lettuce, pat or spin it dry, and tear it into bite-size pieces. Place the lettuce in a large bowl.

4. Make the dressing: Place the garlic, anchovies, tahini, mustard, Worcestershire sauce, and the ½ teaspoon each of salt and pepper in a small bowl and stir them together. Whisk in the lemon juice, water, and the 1½ tablespoons of olive oil.

5. Pour the dressing over the lettuce and toss to coat. Sprinkle the croutons over the salad.

Serves 4

Greek Salad

This Mediterranean salad is one of our favorites and can easily be doubled or tripled for a larger group.

2 cups torn or coarsely chopped iceberg lettuce
½ cucumber, chopped
2 tomatoes, chopped
6 kalamata olives
½ red onion, sliced
¼ cup crumbled light feta cheese
1 tablespoon red wine vinegar
2 teaspoons extra-virgin olive oil
1 teaspoon fresh lemon juice
¾ teaspoon dried oregano
Pinch of salt
Pinch of freshly ground pepper

1. Place the lettuce, cucumber, tomatoes, olives, red onion, and feta in a bowl and toss them together.

2. Place the vinegar, olive oil, lemon juice, oregano, salt, and pepper in a small bowl and whisk them together. Pour the dressing over the lettuce mixture and toss to coat.

Serves 2

Tangy Red and Green Coleslaw

Using a vinaigrette in coleslaw makes it low-fat and really tangy! This is a great keeper salad for the refrigerator or to tote along to a potluck.

4 cups finely shredded green cabbage
2 cups finely shredded red cabbage
2 carrots, shredded
½ cup thinly sliced celery
¼ cup chopped fresh flat-leaf parsley
½ cup cider vinegar
2 tablespoons canola oil
2 teaspoons Splenda
1 teaspoon celery seeds
½ teaspoon salt
Pinch of freshly ground pepper

1. Place the green and red cabbage, carrots, celery, and parsley in a large bowl and toss them together.

2. Place the vinegar, oil, Splenda, celery seeds, salt, and pepper in a small bowl and whisk them together. Pour the vinaigrette over the cabbage mixture and toss to coat.

Serves 4 to 6

Raita Salad

This recipe is based on the refreshing Indian condiment raita. Try serving it with Chicken Curry (see the recipe on page 247).

1 package (11 ounces) baby spinach
1 medium-size English (seedless) cucumber, quartered lengthwise and sliced into ½-inch chunks
2 tomatoes, chopped
½ red onion, thinly sliced
1 cup low-fat plain yogurt
½ teaspoon ground cumin
¼ teaspoon salt

1. Place the spinach, cucumber, tomatoes, and red onion in a large bowl and toss to mix.

2. Place the yogurt, cumin, and salt in another bowl and stir them together. Add the yogurt mixture to the spinach mixture and toss to coat.

Serves 4

Tabbouleh Salad

You often see tabbouleh salad in the grocery store deli, but it's very simple to make at home. The chickpeas add more fiber.

¾ cup bulgur
½ teaspoon grated lemon zest
2 tablespoons fresh lemon juice
2 tablespoons extra-virgin olive oil
1 small clove garlic, minced
½ teaspoon salt
½ teaspoon freshly ground pepper
¼ teaspoon ground cumin
1 can (15½ ounces) chickpeas (garbanzo beans), rinsed and drained
3 plum tomatoes, diced
¼ cucumber, diced
1 cup finely chopped fresh flat-leaf parsley
½ cup finely chopped fresh mint
1 tablespoon chopped fresh chives

1. Bring 1½ cups of water to a boil in a saucepan. Add the bulgur. Cover the pan, reduce the heat to low, and cook until the water is absorbed, about 10 minutes. Using a fork, scrape the bulgur into a large bowl and let cool.

2. Place the lemon zest and juice, olive oil, garlic, salt, pepper, and cumin in a small bowl and whisk them together. Pour the dressing over the cooled bulgur. Add the chickpeas, tomatoes, cucumber, parsley, mint, and chives and stir until well combined.

Serves 4 to 6

Make Ahead: The tabbouleh salad can be refrigerated, covered, for up to 3 days.

Mixed Bean Salad

Packed with fiber, bean salad makes a quick and easy lunch.

1 can (15½ ounces) red kidney beans, rinsed and drained
1 can (15½ ounces) chickpeas (garbanzo beans), rinsed and drained
1 cucumber, chopped
2 tomatoes, chopped
2 cups cooked whole wheat pasta, such as small shells, macaroni, or pasta of a similar size
4 tablespoons chopped fresh flat-leaf parsley
2 tablespoons red wine vinegar
4 teaspoons extra-virgin olive oil
½ teaspoon Dijon mustard
Generous pinch of salt
Generous pinch of freshly ground pepper
Generous pinch of finely chopped fresh herbs, such as thyme or oregano

1. Place the kidney beans and chickpeas in a large bowl and add the cucumber, tomatoes, pasta, and parsley.

2. Place the vinegar, olive oil, mustard, salt, pepper, and herbs in a small bowl and whisk them together. Pour the dressing over the salad and toss to coat.

Serves 4

Cold Noodle Salad with Cucumber and Sesame

These refreshing noodles pair well with Ginger-Wasabi Halibut (see the recipe, page 240).

6 ounces thin pasta, such as vermicelli, capellini, or spaghettini
1 tablespoon rice vinegar
4 teaspoons Splenda
2 teaspoons soy sauce
½ English (seedless) cucumber, quartered lengthwise and thinly sliced
2 teaspoons toasted sesame seeds (see Note)

1. Bring a large pot of salted water to a boil. Cook the pasta until al dente, about 4 minutes. Drain the pasta and rinse it under cold water, then place it in a large bowl.

2. Place the vinegar, Splenda, and soy sauce in a small bowl and stir them together. Pour the dressing over the cooked pasta and stir in the cucumber and sesame seeds; toss to coat well.

Serves 6

Note: To toast the sesame seeds on the stove top, heat them in a frying pan over medium heat until brown and fragrant, 3 to 4 minutes, stirring them occasionally. To toast them in the oven, preheat the oven to 325°F. Spread the sesame seeds out on a rimmed baking sheet and bake them until brown and fragrant, 12 to 15 minutes. Let the sesame seeds cool before using them.

G.I. Pasta Salad

This pasta salad is perfect for taking to work for lunch. It will keep you going all afternoon.

½ to ¾ cup cooked whole wheat pasta, such as spirals, shells, or pasta of a similar size
1 cup chopped vegetables, such as scallions or red onion and cooked broccoli, asparagus, and/or bell peppers
¼ cup light tomato sauce or other low-fat or nonfat pasta sauce
4 ounces cooked chicken or other lean meat, such as lean ground turkey or lean chicken sausage, chopped

Place the pasta, vegetables, tomato sauce, and chicken in a bowl and stir to mix well. Refrigerate the salad, covered, until ready to use, then heat in the microwave or serve chilled.

Serves 1

Variation: You can use the proportions here as a guide: Vary the vegetables, sauce, and source of protein to suit your taste and add variety to your pasta salads.

Crab Salad in Tomato Shells

Big beefsteak tomatoes are ideal here; their size accommodates the filling, and their pulp and seeds are easy to scoop out.

2 cups canned crab
4 large beefsteak tomatoes
¼ cup fat-free mayonnaise
2 tablespoons low-fat sour cream
½ teaspoon grated lemon zest
1 tablespoon fresh lemon juice
2 teaspoons chopped fresh tarragon
Pinch of salt
Pinch of freshly ground pepper
1 cup coarsely chopped canned chickpeas (garbanzo beans), rinsed and drained
½ red bell pepper, diced
¼ cup finely diced celery
¼ cup chopped fresh flat-leaf parsley
2 tablespoons chopped fresh chives
2 tablespoons shredded carrot

1. Place the crab in a fine-mesh sieve and press out any liquid. If necessary, remove and discard any cartilage; set the crab aside.

2. Cut off the top quarter of the tomatoes. Using a small spoon, scoop out and discard the seeds and pulp. Place the tomatoes cut side down on a plate lined with paper towels.

3. Place the mayonnaise, sour cream, lemon zest and juice, tarragon, salt, and ground pepper in a large bowl and stir them together. Add the chickpeas, bell pepper, celery, parsley, chives, and carrot. Add the crab and stir to combine. Divide the crab mixture among the tomatoes, spooning it into the center.

Serves 4

Waldorf Chicken and Rice Salad

Easy to make, and who doesn't love a Waldorf salad, especially a green-light version?

¾ cup cooked basmati or brown rice
1 medium-size apple, chopped
1 or 2 ribs celery, chopped
¼ cup walnuts
4 ounces cooked chicken breast, chopped
1 tablespoon store-bought light buttermilk dressing

Place the rice, apple, celery, walnuts, and chicken in large bowl. Pour the buttermilk dressing on top and stir to mix.

Serves 1

MEATLESS

Fettuccine Primavera

Primavera means springtime in Italian, and you can use your favorite spring vegetables, such as asparagus or fiddleheads, in this pasta. Fortunately, you can get peppers, tomatoes, and peas year-round, so you can make this dish any time.

¼ cup extra-virgin olive oil
2 cups cubed firm tofu
3 cloves garlic, minced
¼ teaspoon red pepper flakes
½ cup vegetable cocktail juice, such as V8
2 cups chopped fresh asparagus, or 2 cups fresh or thawed frozen peas
1 red bell pepper, thinly sliced
1 carrot, thinly sliced
1 yellow zucchini, thinly sliced
6 ounces whole wheat fettuccine or linguine
2 plum tomatoes, chopped
¼ cup chopped fresh flat-leaf parsley
2 tablespoons grated Parmesan cheese

1. Heat 2 tablespoons of the olive oil in a nonstick frying pan over medium-high heat. Brown the tofu on all sides for about 2 minutes. Transfer the tofu to a plate. Reserve the olive oil.

2. Heat the remaining 2 tablespoons of olive oil with the reserved olive oil in a large shallow saucepan over medium heat. Add the garlic and red pepper flakes and cook for 1 minute. Add the vegetable cocktail juice and bring to boil. Reduce the heat and let simmer for 1 minute. Add the asparagus, bell pepper, carrot, and zucchini and cook, stirring, until the vegetables are crisp-tender, about 10 minutes.

3. Meanwhile, bring a large pot of salted water to a boil. Add the fettuccine and cook until al dente, about 8 minutes. Drain the fettuccine and return it to the pot. Add the vegetables and tofu and toss to coat. Stir in the tomatoes, parsley, and Parmesan cheese.

Serves 4

Easy-Bake Lasagna

Though cooking the G.I. way usually means starting from scratch, there are some handy convenience products that are green-light, such as pasta sauce! This lasagna is great for a crowd. Just add a tossed salad.

12 whole wheat lasagna noodles
2 teaspoons canola oil
1 onion, chopped
1 red bell pepper, chopped
8 ounces mushrooms, sliced
¼ teaspoon salt
¼ teaspoon freshly ground pepper
1 package (11 ounces) baby spinach
1½ cups diced firm tofu
1 cup fat-free cottage cheese
⅓ cup liquid egg
1 jar (25 ounces) low-fat pasta sauce
1½ cups shredded part-skim mozzarella cheese
2 tablespoons grated Parmesan cheese

1. Preheat the oven to 350°F

2. Bring a large pot of salted water to a boil. Cook the lasagna noodles until al dente, about 10 minutes. Drain and rinse the noodles under cold water. Lay the noodles flat on damp tea towels and set them aside.

3. Meanwhile, heat the oil in a large nonstick frying pan over medium-high heat. Add the onion, bell pepper, mushrooms, salt, and ground pepper and cook until the vegetables soften and the liquid evaporates, about 8 minutes. Add the spinach and cook, stirring, until wilted, about 2 minutes. Stir in the tofu.

4. Place the cottage cheese and liquid egg in a small bowl, stir them together, then set aside.

5. Ladle ½ cup of the pasta sauce in the bottom of a 13 by 9-inch glass baking dish. Arrange 3 lasagna noodles on top of the sauce. Spread one third of the spinach mixture over the top, then one third of the cottage cheese mixture. Spread another ½ cup of the pasta sauce over the cottage cheese. Sprinkle ⅓ cup of the mozzarella on top. Repeat the layers, ending with noodles on top. Spread the remaining sauce and sprinkle the remaining mozzarella and the Parmesan cheese over the noodles.

6. Cover the baking dish with aluminum foil and bake the lasagna for 45 minutes. Uncover the baking dish and bake until the lasagna is bubbly and a knife inserted in the center is hot to the touch, about 15 minutes. Let the lasagna cool for about 10 minutes before cutting and serving.

Serves 8

Vegetable Crumble

We usually think of a crumble as a dessert, but this one makes a delicious vegetarian main dish or a side dish for meat or fish.

For the crumble

1 tablespoon extra-virgin olive oil
1 cup sliced leeks (white and light green parts only)
1 onion, chopped
1 zucchini, cut into 1-inch pieces (about 1 cup)
1 large carrot, cut into 1-inch pieces (about 1 cup)
1 sweet potato, peeled and cut into 1-inch pieces (about 1 cup)
4 ounces mushrooms, quartered
1 rib celery, sliced into ½-inch pieces (about ¾ cup)
½ red bell pepper, cut into 1-inch pieces
1 tablespoon chopped fresh thyme
¼ cup whole wheat flour
1 cup drained canned plum tomatoes, coarsely chopped
1 cup low-fat, low-sodium vegetable broth
½ cup skim milk
¼ cup chopped fresh flat-leaf parsley
½ teaspoon salt
½ teaspoon freshly ground pepper

For the topping

¼ cup nonhydrogenated soft margarine
¼ cup whole wheat flour
¼ cup wheat bran
¾ cup shredded low-fat cheddar cheese
½ cup chopped mixed nuts
2 tablespoons sesame seeds

1. Preheat the oven to 375°F.

2. Make the crumble: Heat the olive oil in a large saucepan over medium-high heat. Add the leeks and onion and cook until softened, about 5 minutes. Add the zucchini, carrot, sweet potato, mushrooms, celery, bell pepper, and thyme. Cook, stirring often, for 10 minutes. Stir in the ¼ cup of whole wheat flour and cook for 1 minute.

3. Stir in the tomatoes, vegetable broth, milk, parsley, salt, and ground pepper and bring to a boil. Reduce the heat, cover the pan, and let simmer until the vegetables are tender, about 15 minutes.

4. Meanwhile, make the topping: Combine the margarine, the ¼ cup of whole wheat flour, and the wheat bran in a bowl. Then, using your fingers, rub them together until the mixture is crumbly. Stir in the cheddar cheese, nuts, and sesame seeds.

5. Spoon the vegetable mixture into a shallow 8-cup baking dish. Sprinkle the topping over the vegetable mixture, distributing it evenly.

6. Bake the crumble until the topping is crisp and golden and the vegetable mixture is bubbling, about 30 minutes.

Serves 4 to 6

Make Ahead: To make the crumble in advance, add 2 tablespoons of whole wheat flour to the filling in Step 2. After Step 5, cover the crumble well with aluminum foil. It can be frozen for up to 1 month. Bake the crumble straight from the freezer, increasing the cooking time by 1 to 1¼ hours.

Vegetarian Moussaka

Traditionally made with ground lamb, moussaka can be made green-light by using vegetables.

For the eggplant and the tomato sauce

2 large eggplants (about 3 pounds total)
2 teaspoons salt
1 teaspoon canola oil
2 large onions, finely chopped
3 cloves garlic, minced
1 red and 1 green bell pepper, diced
1 tablespoon dried oregano
1 teaspoon ground cinnamon
½ teaspoon freshly ground pepper
¼ teaspoon ground allspice
1 can (28 ounces) diced tomatoes
¼ cup tomato paste
1 can (15½ ounces) chickpeas (garbanzo beans), rinsed and drained
¼ cup chopped fresh flat-leaf parsley

For the cheese sauce

2 tablespoons canola oil
¼ cup whole wheat flour
2 cups warm skim milk
¼ teaspoon salt
Pinch of ground nutmeg
Pinch of freshly ground pepper
⅔ cup liquid egg
½ cup pressed fat-free cottage cheese (see Note)
1 cup crumbled light feta cheese

1. Preheat the oven to 425°F.

2. Prepare the eggplant and the tomato sauce: Cut the eggplants

into slices that are ¼ inch thick and layer them in a colander, sprinkling each layer with some of the 2 teaspoons of salt. Let the eggplant stand for 30 minutes, then rinse the slices and drain them well. Place the sliced eggplant on baking sheets lined with parchment paper and bake them, in batches if necessary, until tender, about 20 minutes. Set the eggplant aside. Reduce the oven temperature to 350°F.

3. Heat the 1 teaspoon of oil in a large, shallow Dutch oven or deep, nonstick frying pan over medium heat. Add the onions, garlic, red and green bell peppers, oregano, cinnamon, the ½ teaspoon of ground pepper, and the allspice and cook until the onions have softened, about 5 minutes. Add the tomatoes and tomato paste and bring to a boil. Add the chickpeas and parsley, reduce the heat, and let the tomato sauce simmer for 15 minutes.

4. Make the cheese sauce: Heat the 2 tablespoons of oil in a saucepan over medium heat. Stir in the flour and cook for 1 minute. Whisk in the milk and cook, whisking gently, until the mixture is thick enough to coat the back of a spoon, about 10 minutes. Stir in the ¼ teaspoon of salt, the nutmeg, and the pinch of ground pepper. Let cool slightly, then whisk in the liquid egg and cottage cheese.

5. Spread one third of the tomato sauce in the bottom of a 13 by 9-inch baking dish. Top it with one third of the eggplant slices and one quarter of the feta cheese. Repeat the layers. After the last layer of eggplant, spread the cheese sauce evenly over the top and sprinkle the remaining feta over it. Bake the moussaka until the top is golden brown, about 1 hour. Let stand for 10 minutes before serving.

Serves 8

Note: For ½ cup pressed cottage cheese, drain ⅔ cup fat-free cottage cheese in a fine-mesh sieve placed over a bowl until all of the excess liquid has been removed.

Bean and Onion Pizza

Here's a restaurant favorite for your G.I. lifestyle.

For the pizza dough

¾ cup warm water
2¼ teaspoons active dry yeast
1¼ cups whole wheat flour, plus up to ¼ cup more, if needed
½ cup wheat bran
Pinch of salt

For the topping

1 teaspoon canola oil
2 onions, thinly sliced
2 cloves garlic, minced
¾ teaspoon finely chopped fresh thyme
Pinch of salt
Pinch of freshly ground pepper
¼ cup sun-dried tomatoes
½ cup boiling water
1 cup canned red kidney beans, rinsed and drained
¾ cup low-fat pasta sauce
2 tablespoons chopped fresh basil
¾ cup crumbled light feta cheese

1. Make the pizza dough: Pour the water into a large bowl and sprinkle the yeast on top. Let stand until frothy, about 10 minutes. Add 1¼ cups of the whole wheat flour and the wheat bran and salt and stir until a ragged dough forms. Let stand, covered, for 30 minutes. Place the dough on a floured surface and knead, adding more of the remaining flour as necessary, just until it forms a soft, slightly sticky dough. Place the dough in a greased bowl, cover it, and let rest until doubled in bulk, about 1 hour.

2. Make the topping: Heat the oil in a nonstick frying pan over medium-high heat. Add the onions and garlic and cook, stirring, until the onions start to turn golden, about 3 minutes. Reduce the heat to medium and add the thyme, salt, and pepper. Continue cooking, stirring occasionally, until the onions are soft and golden brown, about 15 minutes. Set the onions aside.

3. Soak the sun-dried tomatoes in the boiling water for 5 minutes. Drain the tomatoes and discard the liquid. Chop the tomatoes and set aside.

4. Place the beans in a large mixing bowl and, using a potato masher, mash them. Stir in the pasta sauce, sun-dried tomatoes, and basil.

5. Preheat the oven to 425°F.

6. Punch down the dough and roll it out on a floured surface to fit a 12- or 14-inch round pizza pan. Place the dough on the pan, stretching as necessary to fit.

7. Spread the pasta sauce mixture over the pizza dough. Top it with the cooked onion mixture and sprinkle the feta over it.

8. Bake the pizza until golden and crisp, about 20 minutes.

Serves 4

Barley Risotto with Leeks, Lemon, and Peas

Unlike traditional risotto, this barley version doesn't need to be watched or stirred continuously.

1 tablespoon extra-virgin olive oil
½ cup chopped leek
(white and light green parts only)
2 cloves garlic, minced
½ teaspoon chopped fresh thyme
1 cup barley
¼ cup dry white wine or vermouth
3 cups low-fat, low-sodium chicken broth,
plus up to ½ cup more, if needed
1 cup fresh or thawed frozen peas
Zest and juice of 1 medium-size lemon
2 tablespoons grated Parmesan cheese
¼ teaspoon salt
¼ teaspoon freshly ground pepper

1. Heat the olive oil in a saucepan over medium-high heat. Add the leek, garlic, and thyme and cook, stirring, until softened, about 3 minutes. Add the barley and stir until well coated.

2. Add the wine to the pan and stir until it is absorbed. Add the chicken broth and bring to a boil. Cover the pan, reduce the heat to low, and let simmer, stirring occasionally, until the barley is tender, 40 to 45 minutes. If necessary to maintain a creamy consistency, stir in a little more chicken broth or hot water near the end of the cooking time.

3. Stir the peas, lemon zest and juice, Parmesan cheese, salt, and pepper into the barley.

Serves 4 to 6

FISH AND SEAFOOD

G.I. Fish Fillet

You can use virtually any fish in this simple recipe; salmon and trout are favorites in our house. This makes one serving, but you can multiply portions as necessary.

4 ounces fish fillet
1 to 2 teaspoons fresh lemon juice
Pinch of freshly ground pepper

1. Place the fish fillet on a microwave-safe dish and sprinkle the lemon juice and pepper over it. Cover the dish with microwave-safe plastic wrap, folding back one corner slightly to allow steam to escape.

2. Microwave the fish on high power until the fish is opaque and flakes easily when pierced with a fork, 4 to 5 minutes. Let stand for 2 minutes, then serve.

Serves 1

Salmon Pasta

When you can't get to the market for fresh salmon, you can substitute canned salmon—or tuna—instead. Use one 6-ounce can or half of a 14¾-ounce can of salmon or two 3-ounce cans of tuna, preferably low sodium.

2 teaspoons canola oil
1 small onion, finely chopped
2 cloves garlic, minced
2 cups low-fat, low-sodium chicken or fish broth
1 cup whole wheat macaroni
1½ cups chopped broccoli
⅓ cup light herb-and-garlic cream cheese
6 ounces skinless salmon fillet
2 tablespoons chopped fresh flat-leaf parsley
Pinch of salt
Pinch of freshly ground pepper

1. Preheat the oven to 425°F.

2. Heat 1 teaspoon of the oil in a saucepan over medium heat. Add the onion and garlic and cook until softened, about 3 minutes. Add the broth and bring to a boil. Add the pasta and cover the pan. Reduce the heat and let simmer for 10 minutes. Stir in the broccoli and cream cheese. Remove the pan from the heat and let stand, covered, for 10 minutes.

3. Meanwhile, rub the remaining 1 teaspoon of oil on the salmon fillet and sprinkle the parsley, salt, and pepper over it. Place the salmon in a small baking pan and bake until the fish is opaque and flakes easily when pierced with a fork, about 10 minutes. Break the salmon up into chunks and add it to the pasta mixture. Stir gently to combine.

Serves 2

Citrus-Poached Haddock

Citrus fruits and fish are made for each other. This simple dish is impressive enough to serve to company.

1 small onion, finely chopped
1 clove garlic, minced
¼ cup orange juice
¼ cup dry white wine or vermouth
1 teaspoon lemon zest
1 tablespoon fresh lemon juice
¼ cup low-fat, low-sodium fish, chicken, or vegetable broth
1 pound haddock fillet, cut into 4 pieces
2 tablespoons chopped fresh flat-leaf parsley or dill
¼ teaspoon salt
¼ teaspoon freshly ground pepper

1. Place the onion, garlic, orange juice, wine, and lemon zest and juice in a large frying pan and bring to a boil. Boil until the onion is softened and the liquid is reduced by half, about 5 minutes.

2. Add the broth to the frying pan and let come to a boil. Place the haddock in the pan, reduce the heat, and let simmer gently, covered, until the fish is opaque and flakes easily when pierced with a fork, about 10 minutes. Using a slotted spoon, transfer the haddock to a platter and cover to keep warm.

3. Bring the poaching liquid to boil and cook until it is reduced by one third. Stir in the parsley, salt, and pepper. Pour the sauce over the fish.

Serves 4

Ginger-Wasabi Halibut

This fish can also be cooked on the grill. Serve it with Cold Noodle Salad with Cucumber and Sesame (see the recipe on page 223) for a refreshing meal.

2 tablespoons Dijon mustard
2 teaspoons wasabi powder
3 tablespoons mirin or sweet sherry
2 tablespoons minced peeled fresh ginger
2 tablespoons chopped fresh cilantro
1 pound halibut, cut into 4 pieces

1. Preheat the oven to 350°F.

2. Place the mustard and wasabi powder in a bowl and stir them together. Stir in the mirin, ginger, and cilantro. Place the halibut in the marinade and turn to coat. Let stand at room temperature for 20 minutes.

3. Place the halibut on a baking sheet and bake until firm to the touch, 8 to 10 minutes.

Serves 4

Grilled Tuna with Chimichurri Sauce

Traditionally served with Argentinean barbecued beef (*carne asado*), *chimichurri* is also delicious with grilled tuna. This recipe makes extra sauce, which can be served with poultry or meat, or stirred into hot rice.

For the chimichurri sauce

4 cloves garlic, minced
½ red onion, finely chopped
½ red bell pepper, finely chopped
¼ cup chopped fresh cilantro
¼ cup chopped fresh flat-leaf parsley
1 tablespoon chopped fresh oregano
½ cup low-fat, low-sodium vegetable broth
2 tablespoons extra-virgin olive oil
2 tablespoons sherry or red wine vinegar
Pinch of salt
Pinch of freshly ground pepper

For the tuna

4 tuna steaks, about ½-inch thick (4 ounces each)
½ teaspoon salt
½ teaspoon freshly ground pepper

1. Preheat an oiled grill to medium-high.

2. Make the *chimichurri* sauce: Combine the garlic, red onion, bell pepper, cilantro, parsley, and oregano in a bowl. Stir in the vegetable broth, olive oil, sherry, and a pinch each of salt and ground pepper.

(continued)

3. Season the tuna with ½ teaspoon each of salt and ground pepper. Grill the tuna until just charred on the outside and rare in the center, about 2 minutes per side. Serve with a dollop of *chimichurri* sauce on top.

Serves 4

Make Ahead: The *chimichurri* sauce can be refrigerated in an airtight container for up to 5 days.

Pan-Seared Whitefish with Mandarin Salsa

A quick, bright, citrusy salsa lends a tropical note to these hearty fish fillets. You can use tilapia, haddock, or catfish for this elegant meal.

For the mandarin salsa

1 can (14 ounces) no-sugar-added mandarin oranges, drained
1 red bell pepper, diced
½ cup diced cucumber
¼ cup finely diced red onion
3 tablespoons chopped fresh cilantro
1 tablespoon rice vinegar
¼ teaspoon salt
Pinch of freshly ground pepper

For the fish fillets

¾ cup fresh whole wheat bread crumbs
¼ cup chopped fresh flat-leaf parsley
2 tablespoons wheat bran
2 tablespoons wheat germ
1 tablespoon chopped fresh tarragon
¼ teaspoon salt
¼ teaspoon freshly ground pepper
⅓ cup liquid egg
¼ cup whole wheat flour
4 whitefish fillets (4 ounces each)
4 teaspoons canola oil

1. Make the mandarin salsa: Coarsely chop the mandarin oranges and place them in a bowl. Add the bell pepper, cucumber, red onion, cilantro, rice vinegar, the ¼ teaspoon of salt, and the pinch of ground pepper. Toss to combine.

2. Prepare the fish fillets: Prepare 3 large, shallow dishes. In the first, combine the bread crumbs, parsley, wheat bran, wheat germ, tarragon, and the ¼ teaspoon each of salt and ground pepper. In the second, place the liquid egg. In the third, place the whole wheat flour. Dredge a fish fillet in the flour first, shaking off the excess. Coat the fillet with liquid egg, then dredge it in the bread crumb mixture. Repeat with the remaining fillets. Place the prepared fillets on a plate lined with waxed paper and set aside.

3. Heat 2 teaspoons of the oil in a large nonstick frying pan over medium-high heat. Add 2 of the fish fillets and cook, turning once, until golden brown, about 10 minutes. Repeat with the remaining 2 teaspoons oil and fillets. Serve the fish topped with the mandarin salsa.

Serves 4

Thai Red Curry Shrimp Pasta

The combination of curry spices, lime, and cilantro is a hallmark of Thai cooking.

1 pound large raw shrimp, peeled and deveined
1 teaspoon Thai red curry paste
6 ounces whole wheat spaghettini or linguine
1 tablespoon extra-virgin olive oil
4 cloves garlic, minced
2 large tomatoes, peeled, seeded, and chopped
¾ cup dry white wine
Zest and juice of 1 lime
¼ teaspoon salt
¼ teaspoon freshly ground pepper
2 tablespoons chopped fresh cilantro
Lime wedges, for serving

1. Place the shrimp in a bowl and toss it with the curry paste until well coated. Cover the bowl and refrigerate the shrimp for at least 2 hours or up to 8 hours.

2. Bring a large pot of salted water to a boil and cook the pasta until al dente, about 8 minutes.

3. Meanwhile, heat the olive oil in a large nonstick frying pan over medium heat. Add the garlic and cook until it just starts to turn golden, 1 to 2 minutes. Add the tomatoes, wine, lime zest and juice, salt, and pepper and bring to a boil. Reduce the heat and let simmer until the sauce reduces and thickens, about 8 minutes. Add the shrimp and cook, stirring, until it is pink and firm, 3 to 4 minutes. Stir in the cilantro.

4. Drain the pasta and add it to the shrimp mixture, tossing it to coat with the sauce. Serve the pasta with lime wedges.

Serves 4

POULTRY

Chicken Tarragon with Mushrooms

Tarragon adds a light French flavor to chicken. The version here is great for entertaining.

2 teaspoons canola oil
2 skinless, boneless half chicken breasts (4 ounces each)
Freshly ground pepper
1 teaspoon nonhydrogenated soft margarine
1 small onion, chopped
8 ounces mushrooms, sliced
3 tablespoons vermouth or white wine
1 tablespoon chopped fresh tarragon
½ cup low-fat, low-sodium chicken broth or water

1. Heat the oil in a nonstick frying pan over medium-high heat. Sprinkle the chicken with pepper and cook until no longer pink inside, about 6 minutes per side. Transfer the chicken to a plate and cover to keep warm.

2. Add the margarine, onion, and mushrooms to the frying pan and cook, stirring constantly, until the onion is soft, about 5 minutes. Add the vermouth and tarragon and let simmer for 1 minute. Add the chicken broth and let simmer until reduced by half, about 2 minutes. Season with pepper. Serve the sauce over the chicken.

Serves 2

Fried Rice with Chicken

Chinese fried rice is generally high in fat and low in protein and fiber. This low-G.I. version is loaded with chicken and colorful vegetables and won't leave you feeling hungry again soon after eating it.

¾ cup brown rice
Pinch of salt
1½ cups low-fat, low-sodium chicken broth
1 teaspoon Asian (dark) sesame oil
2 skinless, boneless half chicken breasts (4 ounces each), chopped
1 cup sliced mushrooms
1 scallion, chopped
2 carrots, diced
½ cup sliced celery
1 cup canned chickpeas (garbanzo beans), rinsed and drained
¼ cup light soy sauce
2 cups bean sprouts

1. Bring the rice, salt, and 1¼ cups of the chicken broth to a boil in a saucepan. Reduce the heat to low, cover the pan, and cook until the liquid is absorbed, about 25 minutes. Fluff the rice with a fork and set aside.

2. Heat the sesame oil in a large nonstick frying pan over medium-high heat. Add the chicken and mushrooms and cook until the chicken is no longer pink inside, about 8 minutes. Add the scallion, carrots, celery, chickpeas, and cooked rice. Cook, stirring, for 2 minutes to combine.

3. Add the remaining ¼ cup of chicken broth and the soy sauce and cook for 5 minutes. Add the bean sprouts and toss to combine.

Serves 4

Variation: Substitute vegetable broth for the chicken broth and ½ cup of chopped extra-firm tofu for the chicken.

Chicken Curry

Vary the heat and taste of this classic dish by using different kinds or amounts of curry powder.

Vegetable oil cooking spray
(preferably canola or olive oil)
1 medium-size onion, sliced
1 to 2 tablespoons curry powder, or more, to taste
1 cup sliced carrots
1 cup chopped celery
½ cup basmati rice
1 medium-size apple, chopped
¼ cup raisins
2 skinless, boneless half chicken breasts
(4 ounces each), cooked

1. Spray a nonstick frying pan with cooking spray, then place it over medium heat. Add the onion and curry powder, stir to coat the onion with the curry, then cook for 1 minute.

2. Add the carrots and celery, stir to mix, then cook for 1 minute.

3. Add the rice, apple, raisins, and 1 cup of water and stir to mix. Cover the pan, reduce the heat, and let simmer until the liquid is absorbed.

4. Add the cooked chicken and cook until heated through, about 2 minutes.

Serves 2

Chicken Schnitzel

Kids love this dish. You can substitute the more traditional veal scaloppine for the chicken.

4 skinless, boneless half chicken breasts (4 ounces each)
½ cup whole wheat flour
½ teaspoon salt
½ teaspoon freshly ground pepper
2 omega-3 egg whites
½ cup wheat bran
¼ cup wheat germ
¼ cup fine dry whole wheat bread crumbs
1 teaspoon grated orange zest
1 tablespoon extra-virgin olive oil
½ cup fresh orange juice
½ cup low-fat, low-sodium chicken broth
½ cup thinly sliced dried apricots
¼ cup chopped scallions

1. Preheat the oven to 200°F.

2. Using a meat mallet or rolling pin, pound the chicken breasts between 2 pieces of plastic wrap until they are about ¼ inch thick.

3. Combine the whole wheat flour, salt, and pepper in a large, shallow dish or pie plate. Whisk the egg whites in another shallow dish or pie plate. In a third dish or pie plate, combine the wheat bran, wheat germ, bread crumbs, and orange zest.

4. Pat the chicken dry and dredge it in the flour mixture, shaking off the excess. Dip the chicken in the egg whites, letting the excess drip off, then dredge it in the bran mixture, coating it completely.

5. Heat the olive oil in a large nonstick frying pan over medium-high heat. Cook the chicken, working in batches, if necessary, until golden brown and just cooked through, about 4 minutes per side. Transfer the schnitzel to a platter and place it in the oven to keep warm while you make the sauce.

6. In the same frying pan, combine the orange juice, chicken broth, and apricots. Bring to a boil and cook until slightly thickened and syrupy, about 3 minutes. Stir in the scallions. Pour the sauce over the schnitzel.

Serves 4

Spicy Roast Chicken with Tomatoes and Tarragon

This recipe is from our friend Meryle. Serve it with basmati rice or quinoa to soak up the sauce.

4 cups cherry or grape tomatoes, cut in half
5 cloves garlic, peeled and crushed
¼ cup extra-virgin olive oil
2 tablespoons chopped fresh tarragon
2 teaspoons red pepper flakes
4 skinless, boneless half chicken breasts (4 ounces each)
1 teaspoon salt
1 teaspoon freshly ground pepper

1. Preheat the oven to 450°F.

2. Toss the tomatoes with the garlic, olive oil, 1 tablespoon of the tarragon, and the red pepper flakes.

(continued)

3. Place the chicken on a rimmed baking sheet. Arrange the tomato mixture in a single layer around the chicken. Sprinkle the chicken and tomato mixture with the salt and pepper.

4. Bake the chicken until it is no longer pink inside, 30 to 35 minutes. Transfer the chicken to a platter. Spoon the tomatoes and their juices over the chicken and then sprinkle the remaining 1 tablespoon of tarragon on top.

Serves 4

Orange Chicken with Almonds

Fans of sweet-and-sour dishes will surely enjoy this orange-flavored chicken. The almonds add calcium to the dish. Serve the chicken over basmati rice.

2 oranges
1 tablespoon canola oil
2 skinless, boneless half chicken breasts (4 ounces each), diced
2 teaspoons minced peeled fresh ginger
¼ teaspoon salt
¼ teaspoon freshly ground pepper
2 scallions, chopped
1 red bell pepper, chopped
1 green bell pepper, chopped
Pinch of red pepper flakes
¼ cup low-fat, low-sodium chicken broth
3 tablespoons soy sauce
2 teaspoons cornstarch
½ cup sliced almonds, toasted
Steamed basmati rice, for serving

1. Using a rasp or grater, remove 1 teaspoon of zest from one of the oranges and set aside. Cut away the remaining orange peel and pith and discard them. Coarsely chop the orange flesh. Cut the other orange in half and squeeze out its juice; set the juice aside, discarding the orange rind.

2. Heat 1½ teaspoons of the oil in a large nonstick frying pan or wok over medium-high heat. Add the chicken, ginger, and a pinch each of the salt and ground pepper and cook until the chicken is no longer pink inside, about 6 minutes per side. Transfer the chicken to a plate. Add the remaining 1½ teaspoons of oil to the frying pan and cook the scallions, red and green peppers, and red pepper flakes, stirring constantly, until crisp-tender, about 6 minutes.

3. Place the chicken broth, soy sauce, reserved orange zest and juice, cornstarch, and the remaining salt and pepper in a small bowl and whisk them together. Add the chicken broth mixture and the cooked chicken and chopped orange to the frying pan with the vegetable mixture and cook, stirring, until the sauce is thickened and has coated the chicken and vegetables, about 5 minutes. Sprinkle the chicken with the almonds and serve with the rice.

Serves 2

Zesty Barbecued Chicken

The marinade in this recipe helps keep the chicken breasts moist when they are cooked.

¼ cup lemon juice
2 teaspoons chopped fresh rosemary
2 teaspoons canola oil
4 skinless, boneless half chicken breasts (4 ounces each)
⅓ cup Zesty Barbecue Sauce (recipe follows)

1. Place the lemon juice, rosemary, and oil in a bowl and whisk them together. Add the chicken breasts and toss to coat. Let the chicken marinate at room temperature for 30 minutes.

2. Meanwhile, preheat an oiled grill to medium-high.

3. Remove the chicken from the marinade and discard the marinade. Brush the chicken with some of the Zesty Barbecue Sauce, then grill it for 6 minutes. Turn the chicken, brush it with more sauce, and grill it until it is no longer pink inside, about 6 minutes longer.

Serves 4

Zesty Barbecue Sauce

You only need a small amount of this sauce for the barbecued chicken. It will keep for up to two weeks refrigerated in an airtight container. Try it on pork chops, too.

1 can (15 ounces) tomato sauce
2 cloves garlic, minced
¼ cup frozen apple juice concentrate
¼ cup tomato paste
2 tablespoons cider vinegar
1 tablespoon Splenda
1 tablespoon Dijon mustard
2 teaspoons chili powder
½ teaspoon Worcestershire sauce
¼ teaspoon salt
¼ teaspoon freshly ground pepper

Combine the tomato sauce, garlic, apple juice concentrate, tomato paste, vinegar, Splenda, mustard, chili powder, Worcestershire sauce, salt, and pepper in a large saucepan and bring to a boil. Reduce the heat and let simmer, uncovered, until reduced and thickened, about 20 minutes.

Makes about 1½ cups

Rigatoni with Mini Meatballs

For busy families, a little meal preplanning always helps during the week. This hearty casserole can be made ahead of time and frozen for another day.

8 ounces lean ground chicken or turkey
2 tablespoons chopped fresh flat-leaf parsley
1 large clove garlic, minced
1 teaspoon salt
Pinch of freshly ground pepper
1 tablespoon extra-virgin olive oil
1 onion, chopped
2 cups chopped eggplant
1 zucchini, chopped
1 small carrot, finely chopped
1 tablespoon dried oregano
2 cans (28 ounces each) plum tomatoes, pureed
½ cup canned red kidney beans, rinsed and drained
3 cups rigatoni
2 tablespoons grated Parmesan cheese

1. Preheat the oven to 350°F.

2. Place the chicken, parsley, garlic, a pinch of the salt, and the pepper in a bowl and mix until well combined. Using wet hands, roll 1 heaping teaspoon of the chicken mixture into a small meatball and place it on a parchment paper–lined baking sheet. Repeat with the remaining chicken mixture.

3. Bake the meatballs until they are no longer pink inside, about 8 minutes.

4. Meanwhile, heat the olive oil in a large saucepan over medium-high heat. Add the onion and eggplant and cook, stirring, until golden and softened, about 8 minutes. Reduce the heat to medium and add the zucchini, carrot, and oregano. Cook, stirring, until softened, about 5 minutes.

5. Add the pureed tomatoes and the remaining salt and bring to a boil. Add the cooked meatballs and the kidney beans. Reduce the heat and let simmer until the sauce is slightly thickened, about 30 minutes.

6. Meanwhile, bring a large pot of salted water to a boil. Cook the rigatoni until al dente, about 10 minutes. Drain the rigatoni and add it to the meatballs and sauce, stirring to combine. Sprinkle the Parmesan cheese on top.

Serves 4 to 6

Chicken Jambalaya

Jambalaya is a traditional Cajun dish in which rice is used to sop up the rich juices of the stew.

2 teaspoons canola oil
1 onion, chopped
2 ribs celery, chopped
2 cloves garlic, minced
1 pound skinless, boneless chicken breasts, cut into ½-inch cubes
2 teaspoons dried thyme
2 teaspoons dried oregano
1 teaspoon chili powder
¼ teaspoon cayenne pepper (optional)
2 cups low-fat, low-sodium chicken broth
2 green bell peppers, diced
1 can (28 ounces) stewed tomatoes
1 can (15½ ounces) kidney beans, rinsed and drained
¾ cup brown rice
1 bay leaf
¼ cup chopped fresh flat-leaf parsley

1. Heat the oil in a Dutch oven over medium-high heat. Add the onion, celery, and garlic and cook until the onion has softened, about 5 minutes. Add the chicken, thyme, oregano, chili powder, and cayenne, if using, and cook, stirring, for 5 minutes.

2. Add the chicken broth, bell peppers, tomatoes, kidney beans, rice, and bay leaf, and bring to a boil. Reduce the heat to low, cover the Dutch oven, and let simmer, stirring occasionally, until the rice is tender, about 35 minutes. Let stand for 5 minutes. Remove and discard the bay leaf. Stir in the parsley before serving.

Serves 4

MEAT

Beef and Eggplant Chili

The addition of eggplant gives this chili a delicious twist. Sprinkle low-fat Monterey Jack cheese on top for extra zip.

12 ounces extra-lean ground beef
1 tablespoon canola oil
2 onions, chopped
4 cloves garlic, minced
2 tablespoons chili powder
1 tablespoon dried oregano
1 tablespoon ground cumin
2 green bell peppers, chopped
2 cups diced eggplant
1 can (28 ounces) diced tomatoes
½ cup tomato paste
1 can (15½ ounces) red kidney beans, rinsed and drained

1. Brown the beef in a large saucepan over medium-high heat, then transfer it to a plate.

2. In the same saucepan, heat the oil over medium heat. Add the onions, garlic, chili powder, oregano, and cumin and cook, stirring, until the onion is softened, about 5 minutes.

3. Add the green peppers and eggplant and cook until the eggplant is lightly golden, about 10 minutes.

4. Add the tomatoes, tomato paste, and browned beef and bring to a boil. Reduce the heat and add the kidney beans. Let the chili simmer until the eggplant is very tender, about 1 hour.

Serves 4

Horseradish Burgers

Grilled or pan-fried, the combination of beef and horseradish makes these burgers a hit with meat lovers. For a spicier horseradish flavor, simply smother the burgers with more horseradish.

1 small onion, grated
1 clove garlic, minced
2 tablespoons prepared horseradish
2 tablespoons steak sauce
1 tablespoon Dijon mustard
1 tablespoon Worcestershire sauce
2 tablespoons chopped fresh oregano
¼ teaspoon salt
½ teaspoon freshly ground pepper
2 tablespoons wheat bran
2 tablespoons wheat germ
1 pound extra-lean ground beef
2 whole wheat buns, cut in half
4 lettuce leaves
1 tomato, sliced
¼ cup alfalfa sprouts (optional)

1. Place the onion, garlic, horseradish, steak sauce, mustard, Worcestershire sauce, oregano, salt, and pepper in large bowl and stir to mix. Add the wheat bran and wheat germ and stir to coat. Let stand for 5 minutes. Using your hands, mix in the beef until the mixture is well combined.

2. If grilling, preheat an oiled grill to high.

3. Form the meat mixture into 4 patties each about ½ inch thick. Cook the patties on the grill or in a nonstick frying pan over medium heat, turning once, until no longer pink inside, about 12 minutes total.

4. Place each patty on a bun half. Top each patty with a lettuce leaf, tomato slices, and alfalfa sprouts, if using.

Serves 4

Meat Loaf

Serve this meat loaf with new potatoes, green beans, and a salad for dinner.

1½ pounds extra-lean ground beef
1 cup tomato juice
½ cup old-fashioned rolled oats
1 omega-3 egg, lightly beaten
½ cup chopped onion
1 tablespoon Worcestershire sauce
½ teaspoon salt (optional)
¼ teaspoon freshly ground pepper

1. Preheat the oven to 350°F.

2. Combine the beef, tomato juice, oats, egg, onion, Worcestershire sauce, salt, if using, and pepper in large bowl. Mix gently but thoroughly.

3. Press the meat loaf mixture into an 8 by 4-inch loaf pan. Bake until an instant-read meat thermometer inserted into the center registers 160°F, about 1 hour. Let the meat loaf stand for 5 minutes before draining off any juices and slicing it.

Serves 6

Pork Tenderloin with Apple Compote

Serve this comforting dish with Brussels sprouts, sliced carrots, and some boiled new potatoes tossed in lemon juice and parsley.

For the pork

1 tablespoon Dijon mustard
½ teaspoon dried sage
¼ teaspoon dried thyme
Pinch of salt
Pinch of freshly ground pepper
1 pork tenderloin (about 12 ounces)
1 tablespoon canola oil

For the apple compote

1 teaspoon canola oil
2 small apples, cored and diced
1 onion, finely chopped
¼ teaspoon dried thyme
Pinch of salt
Pinch of freshly ground pepper
¼ cup dried currants
2 tablespoons apple juice

1. Preheat the oven to 400°F.

2. Prepare the pork: Place the mustard, sage, thyme, and a pinch each of salt and pepper in a small bowl and stir to mix. Rub the mustard mixture all over the pork tenderloin.

3. Heat the 1 tablespoon of oil in an ovenproof nonstick frying pan over medium-high heat. Brown the pork tenderloin on one side, turn it over, and place the frying pan in the oven until the pork has only a hint of pink inside, about 20 minutes.

4. Meanwhile make the apple compote: Heat the 1 teaspoon of oil in another nonstick frying pan over medium-high heat. Add the apples, onion, thyme, and a pinch each of salt and pepper and cook until light golden, about 5 minutes. Add the currants and apple juice and cook until the apples are crisp-tender, about 1 minute.

5. Let the pork tenderloin stand for 5 minutes before slicing and serving with the apple compote.

Serves 3

Pork Medallions Dijon

Eating the green-light way doesn't mean you have to sacrifice flavor. This pork is fork-tender, and the tasty sauce is rich and creamy.

2 pork tenderloins (about 12 ounces each)
5 tablespoons whole wheat flour
¾ teaspoon salt
¾ teaspoon freshly ground pepper
2 tablespoons extra-virgin olive oil
2 onions, thinly sliced
1 clove garlic, minced
¼ cup Dijon mustard
1¼ cups skim milk
½ cup dry white wine
1 tablespoon chopped fresh tarragon

1. Slice the pork tenderloins crosswise into ¾ inch-thick medallions and place these between 2 pieces of waxed paper. Using a meat mallet or rolling pin, pound the medallions to about a ¼-inch thickness.

(continued)

2. Combine 3 tablespoons of the whole wheat flour and ½ teaspoon each of the salt and pepper on a dinner plate or in a shallow bowl, then dredge the pork in it.

3. Heat 1 tablespoon of the olive oil in a large nonstick frying pan over medium-high heat. Cook the pork until golden brown on both sides, 5 to 7 minutes. Transfer the pork to a plate and cover to keep warm.

4. In same frying pan, heat the remaining 1 tablespoon of olive oil over medium heat. Add the onions and garlic and cook, stirring often, until softened, about 5 minutes. Reduce the heat to medium-low and continue cooking, stirring occasionally, until golden, about 10 minutes longer.

5. Add the remaining 2 tablespoons of whole wheat flour and stir to coat the onion. Add the mustard and cook for 2 minutes. Stir in the milk, wine, and the remaining ¼ teaspoon each of salt and pepper. Cook, stirring constantly, until thickened. (If the mustard mixture is too thick, stir in 1 tablespoon of warm water.) Stir in the tarragon. Return the pork to the pan and cook until heated through, about 1 minute.

Serves 6

Mushroom Gravy Pork Chops

Nothing turns a meal into comfort food better than gravy. For a change, substitute chicken for pork chops.

1 teaspoon dried Italian seasoning
½ teaspoon dried basil
½ teaspoon salt
½ teaspoon freshly ground pepper
4 boneless pork loin chops
2 teaspoons extra-virgin olive oil
1 large onion, thinly sliced
1 pound mushrooms, sliced
1 tablespoon chopped fresh thyme
2 tablespoons whole wheat flour
1 cup low-fat, low-sodium chicken broth

1. Combine the Italian seasoning, basil, and ¼ teaspoon each of the salt and pepper. Sprinkle the seasoning mixture evenly on both sides of the pork chops.

2. Heat the olive oil in a large nonstick frying pan over medium-high heat. Brown the pork chops on both sides, then transfer them to a plate and cover to keep warm.

3. Add the onion, mushrooms, thyme, and the remaining ¼ teaspoon each of salt and pepper to the frying pan. Cook, stirring, for 10 minutes. Sprinkle the whole wheat flour into the pan and cook, stirring, for 1 minute. Pour in the chicken broth, stirring to combine, and bring to a boil. Reduce the heat and let simmer until slightly thickened, about 3 minutes. Return the pork chops to the frying pan and cook, turning occasionally, until just a hint of pink remains inside the pork, about 5 minutes.

Serves 4

SNACKS

Apple Bran Muffins

Ruth created this recipe several years ago when I was trying to lose weight. We would make large batches and freeze them. Then, whenever I needed a snack, I'd warm a muffin in the microwave. They were so convenient and delicious.

¾ cup All-Bran Original or Bran Buds cereal
1 cup skim milk
⅔ cup whole wheat flour
⅓ cup Splenda
2 teaspoons baking powder
½ teaspoon baking soda
¼ teaspoon salt
1 teaspoon ground allspice
½ teaspoon ground cloves
1¼ cups oat bran
⅔ cup raisins
1 large apple, peeled, cored, and cut into ¼-inch cubes
1 omega-3 egg, lightly beaten
2 teaspoons canola oil
½ cup unsweetened applesauce

1. Preheat the oven to 350°F. Line a 12-cup muffin tin with paper or aluminum foil liners.

2. Combine the bran cereal and milk in a bowl. Let stand for a few minutes.

3. Place the whole wheat flour, Splenda, baking powder, baking soda, salt, allspice, and cloves in a large bowl and stir to mix. Stir in the oat bran, raisins, and apple.

4. Combine the egg, oil, and applesauce in a small bowl. Stir the egg mixture and the bran cereal mixture into the dry ingredients. Divide the batter among the muffin cups.

5. Bake the muffins until they are lightly browned and a toothpick inserted in the center of a muffin comes out clean, about 20 minutes.

Makes 12 muffins

Make Ahead: The apple bran muffins can be kept at room temperature for about 2 days or frozen for up to 1 month. (Wrap each muffin individually in plastic wrap and heavy-duty aluminum foil before freezing to help prevent freezer burn. Then, place the muffins in a resealable plastic bag or an airtight container.)

Cranberry Cinnamon Bran Muffins

These muffins are very nutritious, with a high fiber content, and have a great cinnamon flavor.

1 cup wheat bran
½ cup All-Bran Original or 100% bran cereal
¼ teaspoon salt
½ cup boiling water
1 cup skim milk
1 cup dried cranberries
⅓ cup Splenda
1 omega-3 egg
¼ cup canola oil
1¼ cups whole wheat flour
1¼ teaspoons baking soda
1 teaspoon ground cinnamon

1. Preheat the oven to 375°F. Line a 12-cup muffin tin with paper or aluminum foil liners.

2. Combine the wheat bran, bran cereal, and salt in a heatproof bowl. Pour the boiling water on top and stir to combine. Stir in the milk and cranberries and set aside.

3. Whisk the Splenda, egg, and oil together in another bowl. Stir the egg mixture into the bran mixture.

4. Place the whole wheat flour, baking soda, and cinnamon in a large bowl and stir to mix. Pour the bran mixture over the flour mixture and stir until just combined. Divide the batter among the muffin cups.

5. Bake the muffins until a toothpick inserted in the center of a muffin comes out clean, about 20 minutes.

Makes 12 muffins

Make Ahead: The cranberry muffins can be kept at room temperature for about 2 days or frozen for up to 1 month. (Wrap each muffin individually in plastic wrap and heavy-duty aluminum foil before freezing to help prevent freezer burn. Then, place the muffins in a resealable plastic bag or an airtight container.)

Carrot Muffins

These healthful muffins are a delightful source of fiber.

1 cup whole wheat flour
½ cup wheat bran
½ cup ground flaxseed
¼ cup Splenda
2 teaspoons baking powder
½ teaspoon baking soda
2 teaspoons ground cinnamon
1 teaspoon ground ginger
¼ teaspoon salt
1 cup buttermilk
½ cup liquid egg
¼ cup canola oil
1 teaspoon vanilla
1½ cups finely grated carrots
½ cup raisins, softened in hot water for 10 minutes and drained
⅓ cup chopped pecans

1. Preheat the oven to 375°F. Line a 12-cup muffin tin with paper or aluminum foil liners.

2. Combine the whole wheat flour, wheat bran, flaxseed, Splenda, baking powder, baking soda, cinnamon, ginger, and salt in a bowl.

3. Whisk the buttermilk, liquid egg, oil, and vanilla together in a large bowl. Stir in the carrots, raisins, and pecans. Add the flour mixture and stir until just combined. Divide the batter among the muffin cups.

4. Bake the muffins until a toothpick inserted in the center of a muffin comes out clean, 20 to 25 minutes.

Makes 12 muffins

Make Ahead: The carrot muffins can be kept at room temperature for about 2 days or frozen for up to 1 month. (Wrap each muffin individually in plastic wrap and heavy-duty aluminum foil before freezing to help prevent freezer burn. Then, place the muffins in a resealable plastic bag or an airtight container.)

Whole Wheat Fruit Scones

Enjoy these scones with a cup of hot tea. They are even better with a little sugar-free fruit spread.

1½ cups whole wheat flour
½ cup oat bran
½ cup chopped dried apricots or dried cranberries
2 tablespoons Splenda
2 teaspoons baking powder
½ teaspoon salt
¼ teaspoon ground nutmeg
¼ cup nonhydrogenated soft margarine
⅔ cup skim milk
2 tablespoons liquid egg

1. Preheat the oven to 425°F.

2. Combine the whole wheat flour, oat bran, dried apricots, Splenda, baking powder, salt, and nutmeg in a large bowl. Using your fingers, rub the margarine into the flour mixture to combine. Add the milk and toss with a fork to form a soft dough.

3. Place the dough on a floured work surface and knead it gently about 5 times. Pat the dough out to a ½-inch thickness. Using a knife, cut the dough into 8 squares or use a cookie or biscuit cutter to cut out the scones.

4. Place the scones on a baking sheet and brush the tops with the liquid egg. Bake the scones until golden on the bottom, about 12 minutes.

Makes 8 scones

Strawberry Tea Bread

This recipe makes two loaves, one for now and one for the freezer. A slice makes a perfect snack or a delicious dessert paired with sliced berries.

1½ cups whole wheat flour
1½ cups old-fashioned rolled oats
½ cup wheat bran
1 teaspoon cinnamon
1 teaspoon baking soda
½ teaspoon baking powder
½ teaspoon salt
¾ cup liquid egg
¾ cup Splenda
½ cup canola oil
½ cup skim milk
1 teaspoon vanilla
4 cups strawberries, fresh or thawed frozen, mashed

1. Preheat the oven to 375°F. Oil two 9 by 5-inch loaf pans.

2. Place the whole wheat flour, rolled oats, wheat bran, cinnamon, baking soda, baking powder, and salt in a large bowl and stir to mix. Set the dry ingredients aside.

3. Whisk the liquid egg, Splenda, oil, milk, and vanilla together in a separate bowl. Pour the egg mixture over the dry ingredients and stir until just moistened. Stir in the strawberries. Divide the batter evenly between the 2 prepared loaf pans.

4. Bake the tea breads until a toothpick inserted in the center comes out clean, 45 to 50 minutes.

5. Let the tea breads cool in the pans on a rack for 15 minutes. Turn the tea breads out onto the rack and let cool completely.

Makes 2 loaves, 14 to 16 slices each; 1 slice is 1 serving

Make Ahead: The tea breads can be wrapped in plastic wrap or aluminum foil and stored at room temperature for up to 3 days. Or, slice them and wrap each slice in plastic wrap and heavy-duty aluminum foil. You can freeze them for up to 1 month and remove 1-slice portions as desired.

Crunchy Chickpeas

This is an addictive snack with all the crunch and saltiness of chips and pretzels but without the fat!

2 cans (15½ ounces each) chickpeas (garbanzo beans), rinsed and drained
2 tablespoons extra-virgin olive oil or canola oil
½ teaspoon salt
Pinch of cayenne pepper

1. Preheat the oven to 400°F.

2. Place the chickpeas, olive oil, salt, and cayenne in a large bowl and toss to mix. Spread the chickpeas out in a single layer on a large rimmed baking sheet.

3. Bake the chickpeas until golden, about 45 minutes, shaking the baking sheet a couple of times. Let the chickpeas cool completely.

Serves 6

Helpful Hint: Add other spices or more salt to change the flavor of the chickpeas.

DESSERTS

Apple Raspberry Coffee Cake

A piece of this fruit-laden coffee cake makes a delectable light dessert. It can be refrigerated for up to three days.

For the batter

1 cup whole wheat flour
½ cup wheat bran
½ cup Splenda brown sugar
1½ teaspoons baking powder
½ teaspoon baking soda
¼ teaspoon ground cinnamon
¼ teaspoon ground nutmeg
Pinch of salt
½ cup buttermilk
¼ cup nonhydrogenated soft margarine, melted and cooled
¼ cup liquid egg
2 teaspoons vanilla
1 cup fresh raspberries
1 apple, cored and diced

For the topping

⅓ cup old-fashioned rolled oats
¼ cup Splenda brown sugar
2 tablespoons chopped pecans
1 tablespoon nonhydrogenated soft margarine

1. Preheat the oven to 350°F. Line an 8-inch square baking pan with parchment paper.

2. Make the batter: Place the whole wheat flour, wheat bran, ½ cup of Splenda brown sugar, the baking powder, baking soda, cinnamon, nutmeg, and salt in a large bowl and stir to combine. Set the dry ingredients aside.

3. Whisk the buttermilk, melted margarine, liquid egg, and vanilla together in another bowl. Pour the buttermilk mixture over the flour mixture and stir until moistened. Spread two thirds of the batter in the prepared baking pan.

4. Place the raspberries and apple in a bowl and toss them together. Sprinkle the fruit mixture over the batter in the baking pan. Dollop the fruit with the remaining batter, then smooth the batter gently with a wet spatula.

5. Make the topping: Combine the oats, the ¼ cup of Splenda brown sugar, and the pecans and margarine in a bowl. Sprinkle the topping over the coffee cake, pressing it gently into the batter.

6. Bake the coffee cake until a toothpick inserted in the center comes out clean, about 30 minutes.

Makes nine 2-inch-square pieces; 1 piece is 1 serving

Berry Crumble

This is one of my wife, Ruth's favorite green-light desserts. Although it's best made with fresh berries during the summer, it's also lovely made with frozen fruit.

For the filling

5 cups fresh or frozen berries, such as raspberries, blackberries, blueberries, and sliced strawberries
1 large apple, cored and chopped
2 tablespoons whole wheat flour
2 tablespoons Splenda
½ teaspoon ground cinnamon

For the topping

1 cup old-fashioned rolled oats
½ cup chopped pecans or walnuts
¼ cup Splenda brown sugar
¼ cup nonhydrogenated soft margarine, melted
1 teaspoon ground cinnamon

1. Preheat the oven to 350°F.

2. Prepare the filling: Combine the berries and apple in an 8-inch square baking dish.

3. Combine the whole wheat flour, Splenda, and ½ teaspoon of cinnamon in a bowl. Sprinkle the flour mixture over the fruit and toss gently.

4. Make the topping: Combine the oats, pecans, Splenda brown sugar, margarine, and 1 teaspoon of cinnamon in a medium-size bowl. Sprinkle the topping evenly over the fruit mixture.

5. Bake the crumble until the topping is golden and the fruit mixture is bubbling, about 30 minutes.

Serves 6

Plum Crumble

Crumbles are ideal green-light desserts and can be made with a wide array of fruit. Try using 1½ pounds of pears instead of the plums, cutting back slightly on the amount of Splenda.

For the filling

1½ pounds prune plums (such as damson or Italian plums), cut in half and pitted
1 tablespoon Splenda
1 tablespoon cornstarch
½ teaspoon ground ginger
½ teaspoon ground cinnamon

For the topping

¾ cup old-fashioned rolled oats
½ cup whole wheat flour
½ cup Splenda
¼ cup chopped almonds or pecans
¼ cup nonhydrogenated soft margarine
1 teaspoon grated orange zest
½ teaspoon ground cinnamon
¼ teaspoon ground cardamom

1. Preheat the oven to 350°F.

2. Prepare the filling: Place the plums, 1 tablespoon of Splenda, and the cornstarch, ginger, and cinnamon in a bowl and toss to mix. Arrange the plums evenly in a deep 9-inch pie plate.

3. Make the topping: Combine the oats, whole wheat flour, ½ cup of Splenda, and the almonds, margarine, orange zest, cinnamon, and cardamom in a bowl. Using your fingers, rub the ingredients together until a crumbly dough forms. Sprinkle the topping evenly over the fruit mixture.

(continued)

4. Bake the crumble until the topping is golden and the fruit mixture is bubbling, 35 to 40 minutes.

Serves 6

Make Ahead: The crumble can be refrigerated, covered, for up to 2 days.

One-Bowl Chocolate Cake

This delicious cake is green-light when served with fresh berries. You can make a yellow-light version with chocolate ganache icing for a special occasion (see the Variation on the facing page).

1⅓ cups whole wheat flour
¾ cup Splenda
½ cup unsweetened cocoa powder
1½ teaspoons baking soda
1½ teaspoons baking powder
½ teaspoon salt
1 omega-3 egg
1 omega-3 egg white
⅔ cup buttermilk
½ cup unsweetened applesauce
2 tablespoons canola oil
1 teaspoon vanilla
Grated zest of 1 orange

1. Preheat the oven to 350°F. Oil an 8-inch round cake pan or springform pan. Cut a round of parchment paper and line the bottom of the pan.

2. Place the whole wheat flour, Splenda, cocoa powder, baking soda, baking powder, salt, egg, egg white, buttermilk, applesauce, oil, vanilla, and orange zest in a mixer, food processor, or blender and mix just until smooth. Pour the batter into the prepared cake pan and smooth the top.

3. Bake the cake until the top springs back when lightly pressed and a toothpick inserted in the center comes out clean, 20 to 25 minutes.

4. Let the cake cool in the pan on a rack for 30 minutes. Remove the cake from the pan and remove and discard the parchment paper. Let the cake cool completely on the rack.

Serves 8

Ganache Variation: Melt 8 ounces of 70 percent chocolate in a bowl set over barely simmering water. Remove the chocolate from the heat and whisk in 1¼ cups of low-fat soy milk until smooth. Spread the ganache over the top and side of the cake.

Apple Pie Cookies

These cookies combine all the flavors of traditional apple pie and have a texture like a soft granola bar—a great snack.

1 cup old-fashioned rolled oats
¾ cup whole wheat flour
1 teaspoon ground cinnamon
½ teaspoon baking powder
Pinch of ground nutmeg
Pinch of salt
¾ cup unsweetened applesauce
⅓ cup Splenda
⅓ cup liquid egg
2 teaspoons vanilla
1 apple, cored and finely diced

1. Preheat the oven to 275°F. Line a baking sheet with parchment paper.

2. Combine the oats, whole wheat flour, cinnamon, baking powder, nutmeg, and salt in a large bowl.

3. Whisk together the applesauce, Splenda, liquid egg, and vanilla in a separate bowl. Pour the applesauce mixture over the oat mixture and stir to combine. Add the apple and stir to distribute the pieces evenly. Drop the batter by heaping tablespoonfuls onto the prepared baking sheet.

4. Bake the cookies until firm and lightly golden, about 25 minutes. Let cool completely.

Makes about 18 cookies; 1 cookie is 1 serving

Make Ahead: The cookies can be stored in an airtight container for up to 3 days or frozen for up to 2 weeks.

Creamy Lemon Squares

These tiny treats make an ideal midafternoon pick-me-up.

½ cup whole wheat flour
½ cup wheat bran
¼ cup ground almonds
1¼ cups Splenda
¼ cup nonhydrogenated soft margarine
¾ cup liquid egg
2 teaspoons grated lemon zest
½ cup fresh lemon juice
¼ cup buttermilk
2 teaspoons cornstarch
1 teaspoon baking powder

1. Preheat the oven to 350°F. Oil an 8-inch square baking pan.

2. Combine the whole wheat flour, wheat bran, almonds, and ¼ cup of the Splenda in a mixer or food processor. Cut in the margarine until the mixture is crumbly, then press it evenly into the bottom of the prepared pan. Bake until lightly browned, 20 to 25 minutes. Set aside to cool, leaving the oven on.

3. Place the remaining 1 cup of Splenda and the liquid egg in a bowl and whisk them together. Stir in lemon zest and juice, buttermilk, cornstarch, and baking powder. Pour the lemon mixture into the baking pan.

4. Bake the lemon squares until set, 15 to 20 minutes. Let cool to room temperature, then refrigerate for at least 2 hours before cutting into 36 squares (cut 6 evenly spaced strips, then cut each strip into 6 even pieces).

Makes 36 squares; 2 squares are 1 serving

Make Ahead: The lemon squares can be stored in an airtight container for up to 3 days or frozen for up to 1 month.

Pecan Brownies

Brownies, you ask? That's right. These are packed with fiber and are absolutely scrumptious, so get baking! And, no, you most definitely can't taste the beans.

1 can (15½ ounces) white beans, red kidney beans, or black beans, rinsed and drained
½ cup skim milk
⅓ cup liquid egg
¼ cup nonhydrogenated soft margarine, melted
1 tablespoon vanilla
¾ cup Splenda
½ cup whole wheat flour
½ cup unsweetened cocoa powder
1 teaspoon baking powder
Pinch of salt
½ cup chopped toasted pecans

1. Preheat the oven to 350°F. Line an 8-inch square baking pan with parchment paper.

2. Place the beans in a food processor and run the machine until a coarse puree forms. Add the milk, liquid egg, melted margarine, and vanilla and puree until smooth, scraping down the side of the bowl a few times. Set the bean mixture aside.

3. Combine the Splenda, whole wheat flour, cocoa powder, baking powder, and salt in a large bowl. Pour the bean mixture over the flour mixture and stir to combine. Scrape the batter into the prepared pan, smoothing the top. Sprinkle the pecans on top.

4. Bake the brownies until a toothpick inserted in the center comes out clean, about 18 minutes. Let cool on a rack, then cut into 16 squares.

Makes sixteen 2-inch by 1-inch brownies; 1 brownie is 1 serving

Make Ahead: Wrapped in plastic wrap or stored in an airtight container, the brownies will keep for up to 4 days. They can also be frozen for up to 2 weeks.

Part Four

Appendixes

appendix 1:

Results of the e-Clinic

I'M SURE YOU'RE ALL WONDERING HOW EVERYONE DID AFTER the first thirteen weeks of the e-Clinic. Well, I'm really delighted with the participants' overall progress. I'm happy to report that we had a dropout rate of less than 20 percent—and that includes those who had to leave the program for medical reasons, such as chemotherapy and hip replacement. Those who stayed with it lost significant amounts of weight. The results, of course, varied from person to person, but this is in no way a reflection of their commitment or of their achievements—we all have different body shapes, metabolisms, ages, and medical histories and we all lose weight at different rates. They all deserve a big pat on the back!

From Bernadette, who lost 20 pounds and a total of 8 inches from her waist and hips:

> *"I can honestly say that I never felt hungry or deprived during the thirteen weeks. This is probably the most significant and critical difference from other weight-loss approaches that I have tried. Not having to measure and weigh most of the food that I eat has probably been the next most critical factor in the success that I have experienced to*

date. Having to do that in the past with other weight-loss programs and then keep track of points was not compatible with real life and quickly gave way to resentment and failure.

"I do like that the range of choices is so broad in most categories of foods listed and that you don't have a feeling of restriction. . . . I believe that the difference between success at this process of weight loss and failure is quickly overcoming a setback, whether it be making a bad choice or however you want to describe not sticking to the plan. I have come to understand that putting a setback behind you and getting quickly back on track is the key to success. Anything else just perpetuates that 'I blew it and what's the point' feeling and holds you back. . . . I appreciate your support and I am excited about the continued feeling of vitality that I have rediscovered. For that I am very grateful."

From Diane, who lost 19 pounds:

"I am still a little disappointed with my total lost amount, but I know that I am down below what I have been for the past seven years. That is encouraging and I know I will continue the good eating habits I have practiced for the last three months. . . . I think that my husband and I have always practiced pretty good 'home cooking' eating habits—we already used low-fat, sugar-free items and ate lean meats. But I have had a big problem with being a 'stress eater' and a 'social eater' (going out to restaurants, inviting people over, fast-food convenience). You have helped me with these issues a lot! Having items for snacks has also helped me

greatly! . . . I have so much more energy this season than I did a year ago. I can remember last year I didn't even want to put up my Christmas decorations because I just did not have the energy. This year, I feel back to my old self. Now I just need to find that self that I haven't seen since around 1995 (when I was diagnosed with asthma and started gaining my weight back)! I know I can do this—for me! Thanks again! It has been a great three months!"

From Ross, who lost 46 pounds:

"One of the biggest obstacles I personally have found, besides all the usual ones, is poor planning as far as shopping goes. I would run out of green-light items and occasionally revert 'just this once' to red-light foods, as they were quicker because 'I didn't have time to go shopping at the moment and needed to eat.' I now work out a plan for a week or so, listing the days and the meals and a possible menu. . . . This takes only a few minutes to actually do the 'math' and write the list, plus, of course, I have to actually get the shopping done."

From Karen, who lost 16 pounds and a total of 7 inches from her waist and hips:

"My biggest suggestion for others is to have as much green-light food around you as possible for the situations you CAN control. I can control my home and my office (meaning my immediate office, not the communal kitchen). I cannot

control what is available when I am at other people's homes or the office cafeteria, which still serves meat loaf and mashed potatoes or pizza as your two hot choices! I can (however dorky it seems) bring two slices of high-fiber whole wheat bread in my purse, get the insides of my sandwich from the salad bar, and make my own sandwich at the table. Restaurants take practice, but as you've said there are usually enough good choices to cobble together a meal. I've eaten out an average of three lunches and three dinners per week and still have lost weight. Of course, the weeks I brown-bag it and eat dinner at home I have better results.

"I've also learned that I share my home and office with 'diet assassins.' I think they think if they can get me to cheat, it absolves their bad eating habits. Last night I found myself making chocolate chip cookies because my husband and coworkers requested them because '[mine] are the best ever.' As I was dropping the dough onto the cookie sheet I had an epiphany. I told my husband he could bake as many as he wanted, and I wrapped up the rest of the raw dough and brought it in to my coworkers with baking instructions.

"The hardest thing has been adjusting expectations as the weeks wore on. The first few weeks the weight dropped right off me. I was taking the initial weight loss, multiplying by the number of weeks until New Year's Eve, and eyeing a new cocktail dress. No such luck. Things ground to a halt after the eighth or ninth week, with only modest losses. But I'm still down 16 pounds and have either lost a minimal amount or not gained during the holiday season. . . . Rick, thank you for choosing me to be in the group and for your and Ruth's tremendous support during this part of the voyage."

From Kathy, who lost 29 pounds and a total of 19 inches from her waist and hips:

> *"What have I learned over the past thirteen weeks? An enormous amount about myself: that I can say 'no' and mean it, that I can socialize and do okay, that having someone else to share the journey with makes all the difference in the world, that it feels good to accomplish something and see the results beginning to change your thinking and actions, that there is a lot of bad information out there about food and diet that I spent years following and being frustrated with, that I don't have to be hungry or feel like I am being deprived, that I look forward to the weekly weigh-in with positive anticipation rather than negative fear, that whatever happened in childhood is no excuse for being overweight now—what's done is done, forget it, move on! Thank you for opening my eyes to all of this and my mind to accepting it."*

From Pat, who lost 16 pounds:

> *"I am proud of myself this week as I have not only lost more inches, but I am down another pound. . . . What really matters is that the weight continues to drop and I am bound and determined to reach my goal of 140 pounds. . . . As for what tips I can provide, I always ask myself when I think I'm starving, 'Am I hungry, thirsty, or tired?' Also when I am really wanting those red-light foods, I say to myself, 'Do I really need them or want them?' This gets me back on track. I also think about the end result and how I will look and feel. I know that summer is only months away and I want to look fine.*

"When people comment on my weight loss and ask what diet I am on, I inform them this is my new way of eating. I have changed my lifestyle to improve my overall health. . . . I keep using the red leather jacket as motivation. I try it on every Sunday morning to see the progress I have made, and it helps me to stay motivated."

From Nancy, who lost 13 pounds and over 10 inches from her waist and hips:

"Gosh, sometimes this is such a mental struggle! Like many people, I've used food as a source of comfort over the years, particularly sweets. I spent two days in the hospital this week (asthma), so I felt sorry for myself and let myself eat things I know better than to eat—what's up with that? It's so frustrating.

"I think it's a mind-set thing, in that I need to get back to the place where I simply choose not to eat sweets, where it's not even an option, let alone a desire. Does that make sense? I've reached that place with fried foods, in that I physically cannot handle eating anything fried anymore. I want to reach that same place with sweets, though admittedly they've had a much stronger 'hold' over me than fried foods ever did.

"Ah well, it's a journey and I press on. Besides, I have to remember that not only am I working toward losing weight and regaining my physical health, but I'm also sorting through a lot of long-standing mental attitudes at the same time. It's all part of the long-term success, I think, in that I have to deal with all aspects of the weight gain, not just the physical."

Congratulations, everyone!

appendix 2:

The Complete G.I. Diet Food Guide

Beans			
	Baked beans with pork Fava beans Refried beans	Kidney beans (canned) Lentils (canned)	Baked beans (low-fat, ½ cup) Black beans Black-eyed peas Butter beans Chickpeas Italian beans Kidney beans Lentils Lima beans Mung beans Navy beans Peas Pinto beans Refried beans (low-fat) Romano beans Soybeans Split peas

Beverages

	Alcoholic drinks Coconut milk Fruit drinks Milk (whole or 2%) Regular coffee Regular soft drinks Rice milk Sweetened juice Watermelon juice	Coffee (with skim milk, no sugar) Diet soft drinks (with caffeine) Milk (1%) Most unsweetened juice Red wine (one glass, preferably with dinner) Vegetable juice	Bottled water Club soda Decaffeinated coffee Diet, caffeine-free soft drinks Herbal tea Light instant hot chocolate Milk (skim) Soy milk (plain, low-fat) Tea

Breads

	Bagels and rolls Baguettes and other crusty white breads Cakes and cookies Cornbread Crispbreads (regular) Croissants and pastries Croutons English muffins Hamburger/hot dog buns Kaiser rolls Melba toast Muffins/doughnuts Pancakes/waffles Pizza Stuffing Tortillas White bread	Crispbreads with added fiber Pita (whole wheat) Sourdough bread Tortillas (whole wheat) Whole-grain breads	100% stone-ground whole wheat bread* High-fiber crispbreads* Whole-grain, high-fiber breads (3g fiber per slice)*

*Limit serving size (see page 20).

Cereal

	All cold cereals except those listed as yellow- or green-light Cereal/granola bars Cream of Wheat Granola Instant/Quick-cook oatmeal Muesli (commercial)	Kashi Golean Crunch! Kashi Good Friends Shredded Wheat 'N Bran	100% bran cereals (such as All-Bran) Cold cereals with at least 10g fiber per serving Kashi Golean Oat bran Oatmeal/porridge (old-fashioned rolled oats or steel-cut oats)

Cereal Grains

	Amaranth Almond flour Couscous Millet Polenta Rice (short-grain, white, instant) Rice cakes Rice noodles	Cornstarch Spelt Whole wheat couscous	Arrowroot flour Barley Buckwheat Bulgur Gram flour Kamut (not puffed) Quinoa Rice (basmati, brown, long-grain, wild) Wheat berries

Condiments and Seasonings

	Ketchup Mayonnaise Tartar sauce	Mayonnaise (light)	Capers Chili powder Extracts (vanilla, etc.) Garlic

Condiments and Seasonings *(continued)*

			Gravy mix (maximum 20 calories per ¼ cup serving) Herbs Horseradish Hummus Mayonnaise (fat-free) Mustard Salsa (sugar-free) Sauerkraut Soy sauce (low sodium) Spices Teriyaki sauce Vinegar (all types) Worcestershire sauce

Dairy

	Almond milk Cheese Chocolate milk Coconut milk Cottage cheese (whole or 2%) Cream Cream cheese Evaporated milk Goat milk Ice cream Milk (whole or 2%) Rice milk	Cheese (low-fat) Cream cheese (light) Frozen yogurt (low-fat, low-sugar) Ice cream (low-fat) Milk (1%) Sour cream (light) Yogurt (low-fat, with sugar)	Buttermilk (skim/1%) Cheese (fat-free) Cottage cheese (1% or fat-free) Cream cheese (fat-free) Extra-low-fat cheese (e.g., Laughing Cow Light, Boursin Light) Fruit yogurt (fat-free, with sweetener)

(continued)

Dairy *(continued)*			
	Sour cream Yogurt (whole or 2%)		Ice cream (½ cup, low-fat and no added sugar) Milk (skim) Sour cream (fat-free) Soy milk (plain, low-fat) Soy cheese (low-fat) Whey protein powder

Fats & Oils			
	Butter Bottled salad dressings Coconut oil Hard margarine Lard Mayonnaise Palm oil Peanut butter (regular and light) Tropical oils Vegetable shortening	Corn oil Bottled salad dressings (light) Mayonnaise (light) Most nuts Natural nut butters Natural peanut butter (no sugar added) Peanuts Peanut oil Pecans Sesame oil Soft margarine (non-hydrogenated) Soy oil Sunflower oil Vegetable oils Walnuts	Almonds* Canola oil* Cashews* Flaxseed Hazelnuts* Macadamia nuts* Mayonnaise (fat-free) Olive oil* Pistachios* Salad dressings (low-fat, low sugar) Soft margarine (non-hydrogenated)* Vegetable oil sprays Vinaigrette

*Limit serving size (see page 20).

Fruits			
Fresh	Cantaloupes Honeydew melons Kumquats Watermelons	Apricots Bananas Custard apples Figs Kiwis Mangoes Papayas Persimmons Pineapples Pomegranates	Apples Avocado (¼) Blackberries Blueberries Cherries Cranberries Grapefruit Grapes Guavas Lemons Nectarines Oranges Peaches Plums Pears Raspberries Rhubarb Strawberries
Bottled, Canned, Dried, Frozen	All canned fruit in syrup Applesauce containing sugar Most dried fruit (including dates and raisins)	Canned apricots in juice or water Dried apples Dried apricots* Dried cranberries* Fruit cocktail in juice	Applesauce (no sugar added) Frozen berries Fruit spreads (extra fruit/ no sugar added) Mandarin oranges Peaches/pears in juice or water

Juices			
	Fruit drinks Prune juice	Apple juice (unsweetened)	Eat the fruit rather than drink its juice

(continued)

*Use sparingly.

Juices *(continued)*			
	Sweetened juice Watermelon juice	Cranberry juice (unsweetened) Grapefruit juice (unsweetened) Orange juice (unsweetened) Pear juice (unsweetened) Pineapple juice (unsweetened) Vegetable juice	

Meat, Poultry, Fish, Eggs, and Tofu			
	Beef (brisket, short ribs) Bologna Breaded fish and seafood Duck Fish canned in oil Goose Ground beef (more than 10% fat) Hamburgers Hot dogs Lamb (rack) Organ meats Pastrami (beef) Pâté Pork (back ribs, blade, spareribs) Regular bacon Salami	Beef (sirloin steak, sirloin tip) Chicken or turkey legs (skinless) Corned beef Dried beef Flank steak Ground beef (lean, 6–10% fat) Lamb (fore/leg shank, center cut loin chop) Pork (center loin, fresh ham, shank, sirloin, top loin) Tofu Turkey bacon Whole omega-3 eggs	All fish and seafood (fresh, frozen, or canned in water) Beef (top/eye round steak) Canadian bacon Chicken or turkey breast (skinless) Egg whites Ground beef (extra lean, 5% or less fat) Lean deli ham Liquid eggs Moose Pastrami (turkey) Pork tenderloin Rabbit Sashimi Soy/whey protein powder

Meat, Poultry, Fish, Eggs, and Tofu *(continued)*			
	Sausages Sushi Whole regular eggs		Soy cheese (low-fat) Tofu (low-fat) Turkey roll TVP (textured vegetable protein) Veal Veggie burgers Venison

Pasta			
	All canned pastas Gnocchi Macaroni and cheese Noodles (canned or instant) Pasta filled with cheese or meat Rice noodles		Dried pasta of any shape, cooked al dente* Mung bean noodles Whole wheat pasta*

Pasta Sauces			
	Alfredo Canned/bottled sauces with added meat or cheese Canned/bottled sauces with added sugar or sucrose	Canned/bottled sauces with vegetables (no added sugar)	Canned/bottled sauces with vegetables (light, no added sugar, e.g., Healthy Choice) Homemade green-light sauces

*Limit serving size (see page 20).

Snacks			
	Bagels Candy Cookies Crackers Doughnuts Flavored gelatin (all varieties) French fries Ice cream (full-fat) Muffins Popcorn (microwaved or pre-popped) Potato chips Pretzels Pudding Raisins Rice cakes Sorbet Tortilla chips Trail mix White bread	Bananas Dark chocolate (70% cocoa) Ice cream (low-fat) Most nuts Popcorn (air popped)	Almonds* Applesauce (unsweetened) Canned peaches/ pears in juice or water Cottage cheese (1% or fat-free) Extra-low-fat cheese (e.g., Laughing Cow Light, Boursin Light) Fruit yogurt (fat-free with sweetener) Nutrition bars (½ bar) Hazelnuts* Homemade green-light snacks (see pp. 264–271) Ice cream (low-fat and no added sugar) Most fresh fruit Most fresh vegetables Most seeds (flax, sesame, sunflower) Pickles Soy nuts Sugar-free hard candies

*Limit serving size (see page 20).

Soups			
	All cream-based soups Canned black bean Canned green pea Canned pureed vegetable Canned split pea	Canned chicken noodle Canned lentil Canned tomato	Chunky bean and vegetable soups (e.g., Campbell's Healthy Request, Healthy Choice) Homemade soups with green-light ingredients (see pp. 211–214)

Spreads and Preserves			
	All products that have sugar as the first ingredient listed		Fruit spreads (extra fruit, no sugar added)

Sugar and Sweeteners			
	Corn syrup Glucose Granulated sugar (all types) Honey Molasses	Fructose Sugar alcohols (e.g., maltitol, xylitol)	Aspartame Equal Splenda Stevia (note: not FDA approved) Sugar Twin Sweet'N Low

Vegetables			
	Fava beans French fries Hash browns Parsnips Potatoes (instant)	Artichokes Beets Corn Potatoes (boiled) Pumpkin	Alfalfa sprouts Asparagus Beans (green/wax) Bell peppers Bok choy

(continued)

Vegetables *(continued)*			
	Potatoes (mashed or baked) Rutabagas Turnips	Squash Sweet potatoes Yams	Broccoli Broccoli rabe Brussels sprouts Cabbage (all varieties) Carrots Cauliflower Celery Collard greens Cucumbers Eggplant Fennel Hearts of palm Hot peppers Kale Kohlrabi Leeks Lettuce Mushrooms Mustard greens Okra Olives* Onions Peas Pickles Potatoes (boiled, new or small)* Radicchio Radishes Snow peas Spinach Swiss chard Tomatoes Zucchini

*Limit serving size (see page 20).

Indexes

General Index

Also see the Recipe Index on pages 315–21.

A

Abdominal fat, 41, 153–54
Activities:
  as distraction from cravings, 87
  as substitute for unconscious or emotional eating, 120–21
  see also Exercise
Aerobic exercise, 171, 172
  indoor activities for, 175–76
  outdoor activities for, 173–75
Alcohol:
  cocktail parties and, 160
  in Phase I, 38
  in Phase II, 195–96
  wine, 66, 195
Almonds, 8
Alzheimer's disease, 7, 37, 54, 153
American College of Rheumatology, 154
American Institute for Cancer Research, 152
Anger, emotional eating and, 118, 120
Antioxidants, 3
  in tea, 24, 37–38
Anxiety:
  about starting diet, 55–56
  caused by weight loss, 183–88
Appearance:
  as motivator to lose weight, 53
  see also Body image
Apple juice, 38
Arby's, 100
Arterial system, 7, 150, 151
Arthritis Care & Research, 154
"At-risk" situations, 119
Automatic behaviors, 119

B

Bacon, 27
Bad habits:
  breaking, 74–80
  emotional, to watch out for, 119–20
  top ten, 75–80
Baked goods, 5
  in G.I. Diet Clinic pantry, 47
Baking ingredients, in G.I. Diet Clinic pantry, 47
Balanced lives, role of food in, 117
Barley, 5
Beans and legumes, 3, 5, 8, 9, 12, 33, 66
  filling your plate and, 20–21
  G.I. Diet Food Guide for, 290
Beef:
  low-fat cuts of, 32
  steaks, 32, 197
  see also Meat, red
Behavior change, 73–80, 119–21
  and emotional bad habits to watch out for, 119–20
  gradual modification and, 120
  rewards for, 56, 119
  substitute activities and, 120–21
  top ten bad habits and, 75–80
Beverages, 36–38
  alcoholic, 38, 66, 160, 195–96
  to avoid, 36, 38
  best green-light choices, 37–38
  cocktail parties and, 160, 195–96
  coffee, 24–25, 36, 37, 57–58, 96, 196
  G.I. Diet Food Guide for, 291
  juices, 36, 196, 295–96
  not drinking enough, 77–78
  teas, 24, 37–38
  water, 37, 77–78, 95
Bicycling. *See* Cycling
Birthdays, 96, 102
Blood pressure, high, 44, 150–51
Blood sugar:
  alcohol and, 38

cravings and, 87
glycemic index and, 10–14
insulin and, 12–13, 24, 75, 131, 142
menopause and, 131
skipping breakfast and, 75
$10 cure and, 142–43
withdrawal symptoms and, 57
see also Glucose
Body image:
and anxiety caused by weight loss, 185, 186–88
negative, 118, 187–88
positive, 53
Body mass index (BMI), 15–18
table for, 16–17
weight-loss target and, 40–42
Boredom, emotional eating and, 118, 120
Bowel function, 5
Brain, protein as critical food for, 8
Bran, 66
Breads, 3, 5
dining out and, 95
G.I. Diet Food Guide for, 291
in Phase II, 196, 197
for sandwiches, 31
serving size for, 20
for toast, 25
Breakfast, 21–27
bacon in, 27
butter and jams in, 26
cereals in, 25, 76, 94, 196
coffee and tea in, 24–25, 57–58, 196
dairy products in, 26
eating out while traveling and, 94
eggs in, 26
G.I. Diet Clinic pantry and, 47
importance of, 21
in Phase II, 196
recipes for, 202–10
red-, yellow-, and green-light foods for (charts), 22–24
skipping, 8, 75
toast in, 25
Breast cancer, 7
Broiling, 32
Brown-bag lunches, 30
Brown sugar, substitute for, 67
Buddies, weight-loss, 140–42
Burger King, 99
Business functions, eating at, 103–4
Butter, 26, 66

C

Caffeine, 24, 36, 37, 96
in Phase II, 196
withdrawal symptoms and, 57–58
Calories:
in alcoholic beverages, 38
excessive consumption of, 2
expended in exercise, 3
in fats, 6, 8
food labels and, 43–44
in fruits and vegetables vs. juices, 36
Canadian bacon, 27, 196
Cancer, 54
abdominal fat and, 41, 154
carbohydrates and, 3
saturated fats and, 7, 152
Candy, 80
Canned foods:
in G.I. Diet Clinic pantry, 47
sodium in, 45
Canola oil, 8, 20, 66
Carbohydrates, 2, 3–5, 9
for breakfast, red-, yellow-, and green-light choices (charts), 22–23
digestive process and, 3–4, 10, 11
fiber in, 3, 5. *See also* Fiber
filling your plate and, 20–21
glycemic index and, 10–14
for lunch and dinner, red-, yellow-, and green-light choices (charts), 28–29
processed foods and, 4–5
in snacks, 35
Celebrations, 79–80, 159–63
alcohol and, 160, 195–96
see also Holidays
Cereal, 4, 5, 25, 44, 76, 94
before dining out, 95
G.I. Diet Food Guide for, 292
in Phase II, 196
serving size for, 20

Changing behaviors. *See* Behavior change
Cheeses, 47, 66
Chicken, 32
  see also Poultry
Childhood, origins of emotional eating in, 118–19
Children, parents' behavior as influence on, 121
Chocolate, 87–88
  in Phase II, 195, 196, 197
Cholesterol:
  fiber and, 5
  HDL and LDL, 7, 151
  monounsaturated fats and, 8
  omega-3s and, 8
  as risk factor for heart disease and stroke, 7, 150, 151
Citrus fruits, 5
Cleaning your plate, 78–79, 118–19
Clothing, as motivator to lose weight, 53, 138, 139
Club soda, 37, 160
Cocktail parties, 160, 195–96
Coconut oil, 7
Cod, 33
Coffee, 24–25, 36, 37, 96
  in Phase II, 196
  withdrawal symptoms and, 57–58
Colorectal cancer, 7, 152
Comfort, using food for, 117–23
  see also Emotional eating
Commute, incorporating walking into, 173
Condiments, 47
  G.I. Diet Food Guide for, 292–93
Congestive heart failure, 150
Convenience foods, 75–76
Cooking ahead, 67
Cooling down, 172
Corn, 197
Cornflakes, 4
Corn oil, 7
Corn syrup, 44, 66
Cottage cheese, low-fat, 26
Cranberry sauce, 162
Cravings, dealing with, 87–88
Cycling, 170, 171, 174–75
  on stationary bike, 175–76

D

Dairy products, 3
  in breakfast, 26
  full-fat, 9, 26
  G.I. Diet Food Guide for, 293–94
  in G.I. Diet Clinic pantry, 47
  low-fat, 9, 12, 26, 34–35, 67, 80
  as protein source, 8, 9
Dehydration, 77–78
Deli foods, in G.I. Diet Clinic pantry, 47
Dementia, 24
Desserts, 34–35
  dining out and, 96
  holiday dinners and, 161, 162
  recipes for, 272–81
  red-, yellow-, and green-light foods for (charts), 35–36
Dextrose, 44
Diabetes:
  exercise and, 170
  glycemic index and, 10–11
  risk factors for, 41, 54, 80, 151–52
Diabetes Dialogue, 152
Diets, reasons for failure of, vii, viii, 55–56
Diet sodas, 37
Digestion:
  carbohydrates and, 3–4, 10, 11
  fats and, 6
  proteins and, 8, 9, 67
Dining out. *See* Eating out
Dinner, 27–30, 31–34
  in Phase II, 197
  potatoes, pasta, or rice in, 34
  protein options in, 32–34
  red-, yellow-, and green-light foods for (charts), 27–30
  vegetables in, 34
Disappointment, with slow rate of weight loss, 109–12
Distracting yourself, from cravings, 87
Doctors, consulting, before starting G.I. Diet, 39–40

Drinks. *See* Beverages
Duck, 96

E

Eating:
  slowly vs. quickly, 77, 95, 120
  unconsciously, 77, 120–21
Eating out, 93–104
  breads or rolls and, 95
  at business functions, 103–4
  eating slowly and, 95
  serving sizes and, 93–94, 96
  soups or salads and, 95–96
  taking edge off appetite before, 95
  top ten tips for, 95–96
  traveling and, 94
  vegetables rather than starchy sides in, 96
  see also Fast food
e-Clinic:
  monthly e-letters and, 198–99
  origins of, viii–x
  results of, 284–89
  weekly sequence of, x–xi
Eggs, 8, 26
  filling your plate and, 20–21
  G.I. Diet Food Guide for, 296–97
  liquid, 8, 9, 26
  with omega-3, 8
Elliptical walkers, 176
Emotional eating, 117–23
  becoming conscious of your eating habits and, 119–20
  changing behaviors and, 119
  childhood origins of, 118–19
  feelings leading to, 118
  and habits to watch out for, 119–20
  substituting pleasurable activities for, 120–21
Energy:
  burned by muscles, 177
  carbohydrates as source of, 3–4
  exercise and, 169
  extra, stored as fat, 6, 12
  increased level of, as reason to lose weight, 53–54, 139
Estrogen, 130, 131
Exercise, 3, 54, 169–78
  aerobic, 171, 172
  benefits of, 170
  indoor activities, 175–78
  lack of, as health risk, 150, 151
  outdoor activities, 173–75
  rewarding yourself with food after, 78
  strength (resistance) training, 171–72, 176–77
  stretching, 172
  weight loss and, 78, 170–71

F

Falling off the wagon, 85–88
  cravings and, 87–88
Family:
  dispiriting comments from, 184, 185
  support from, 140, 141
Fast food, 2, 5, 97–102
  Arby's, 100
  Burger King, 99
  ground rules for, 97
  KFC, 101
  McDonald's, 98–99
  Quiznos, 101–2
  sodium in, 45
  Subway, 98
  Taco Bell, 100
  $10 cure and, 142–43, 194
  Wendy's, 100
Fat, body:
  abdominal, 41, 153–54
  body mass index (BMI) and, 15–18
  energy reserves stored as, 6, 12
Fats, dietary, 2, 3, 6–8, 9
  adapting your standby recipes and, 66
  "bad" and "really ugly," 7, 9
  for breakfast, red-, yellow-, and green-light choices (charts), 24
  calories in, 6, 8
  digestive process and, 6
  filling your plate and, 20–21
  food labels and, 44
  G.I. Diet Food Guide for, 294
  "good" and "best," 7–8
  health risks associated with, 7, 152, 153

LDL levels and, 151
for lunch and dinner, red-, yellow-, and green-light choices (charts), 30
saturated, minimizing in red meat, 32
weight loss and, 6–7
Feelings:
caused by weight loss, 183–88
see also Emotional eating
Fiber, 3, 5, 9
adapting your standby recipes and, 66
in beans and legumes, 33
boosting, 66
food labels and, 44
in fruits and vegetables vs. juices, 36
processing or cooking foods and, 14
taking edge off appetite and, 95
Filling your plate, 20–21
at holiday dinners, 161
Fish and seafood, 8, 9, 33, 67
filling your plate and, 20–21
G.I. Diet Food Guide for, 296–97
recipes for, 237–44
in restaurants, 96
serving size for, 20
Fitness clubs, 170–71, 175
Flavonoids, 37–38
Flaxseed, 8
Fletcher, Horace, 77
Flexibility, stretching and, 172
Flour, white, 5
Folic acid, 34
Food guide. *See* G.I. Diet Food Guide
Freezing meal-sized portions, 67
Friends, support from, 140–42
Fructose, 44
Fruit, 3, 12, 34, 76, 94, 96
blood pressure and, 150–51
G.I. Diet Food Guide for, 295
in G.I. Diet Clinic pantry, 46
as snack, 35, 76, 80
Fruit juices, 36, 196
G.I. Diet Food Guide for, 295–96
Fruit spreads, 26

G

Gallop, Ruth, 117–21
G.I. *See* Glycemic index
G.I. Diet, 15–47
assessing whether it's right time to start, 40
consulting doctor or health care practitioner before starting, 39–40
creation of, vii–viii
getting ready to start, 39–45
meal basics for, 21–38
nutritional basis for, 2–14
setting weight-loss target for, 40–42
starting with Preliminary Phase or Phase I, 15, 18–19
when and how much to eat in, 19–21
G.I. Diet Clinic:
pantry for, 46–47
Week 1, 50–62
Week 2, 63–72
Week 3, 73–84
Week 4, 85–92
Week 5, 93–108
Week 6, 109–16
Week 7, 117–28
Week 8, 129–36
Week 9, 137–48
Week 10, 149–58
Week 11, 159–68
Week 12, 169–82
Week 13, 183–92
Week 13, beyond (Phase II), 193–99
see also e-Clinic
G.I. Diet Food Guide, 290–300
beans, 290
beverages, 291
breads, 291
breakfast choices, 22–24
cereal, 292
condiments and seasonings, 292–93
dairy products, 293–94
dessert and snack choices, 35–36
fats and oils, 294
fruits, 295
grains, 292
juices, 295–96
lunch and dinner choices, 27–30
meat, poultry, fish, eggs, and tofu, 296–97
pasta, 297

pasta sauces, 297
snacks, 298
soups, 299
spreads and preserves, 299
sugar and sweeteners, 299
vegetables, 299–300
Glucose, 44
carbohydrates broken down into, 3–4, 5, 10, 11
glycemic index and, 10–14
see also Blood sugar
Glycemic index (G.I.), 10–14
examples of ratings in, 11
red-, yellow-, and green-light categories in, 13–14
Goals:
mini-, setting, 56
see also Target weight
Grains, 3, 5
G.I. Diet Food Guide for, 292
in G.I. Diet Clinic pantry, 47
whole, 5, 12, 66
Grazing, 76, 119
Green-light foods, xi, 13–14
adapting your standby recipes and, 66
carrying as emergency reserves, 94
filling your plate with combination of, 20–21
pantry guide, 46–47
satisfying cravings with, 87
serving sizes for, 19–20
shopping for, 43–45
Grilling, 32
Grocery lists, 43
for each week of G.I. Diet Clinic, 43, 64. *See also specific weeks*

H

Habits. *See* Bad habits
Ham, 27
Hamburgers, fast-food, 97
$10 cure and, 142–43, 194
HDL, 7, 151
Health improvements, as reason to lose weight, 54, 139
Health risks, of excess weight and poor diet, 54, 149–54
abdominal fat and, 41, 153–54
Alzheimer's disease and, 7, 54, 153
cancer and, 7, 54, 152
diabetes and, 54, 151–52
heart disease and stroke and, 7, 41, 44, 54, 80, 149–51, 154
hypertension and, 44, 150–51
joint degeneration and, 154
Heart attack, 7, 150
Heart disease:
abdominal fat and, 41, 154
antioxidants and, 3, 24, 37
carbohydrates and, 3
exercise and, 170
monounsaturated fats and, 8
red wine and, 195
risk factors for, 7, 41, 44, 54, 80, 149–51, 154
Heart health, omega-3s and, 8, 33
Heart rate, exercise and, 173, 174
Herbal teas, 24, 38, 78
Herbs, 47
High blood pressure, 44, 150–51
Hiking, 171, 174, 176
Hip measurements:
recording each week, 50–51
waist-to-hip ratio and, 154
Hip replacements, 154
Holidays, 159, 160–63
dinners at someone else's home and, 160–61
high-sugar, high-fat treats and, 79–80
hosting dinner at your own home and, 161–62
Home gyms, 175–76, 177
Hunger, 19
caffeine and, 24, 36
processed foods and, 4–5
shopping and, 42–43, 79
Hydrogenated oils, 7, 44
Hypertension, 44, 150–51

I

Inactivity, as risk factor, 150
Indoor activities, as exercise, 175–78
Insoluble fiber, 5, 66

Insulin, 12–13, 75, 131, 142
caffeine and, 24, 36
Irritability, emotional eating and, 118, 120

J

Jams, 26
Jenkins, David, 10
Jogging, 171, 173–74, 176
Joint degeneration, 154
Juices, 36, 196
G.I. Diet Food Guide for, 295–96

K

KFC, 101
Kitchen, green-light makeover in, 42
Knee replacements, 154

L

Labels, reading, 43–45
LDL, 7, 151
Legumes. *See* Beans and legumes
Loneliness, emotional eating and, 118, 120
Looking better, as reason to lose weight, 53
"Low-fat" foods, 35, 44
Lunch, 27–31
brown-bagging, 30
in Phase II, 197
red-, yellow-, and green-light foods for (charts), 27–30

M

Maintaining weight loss:
exercise and, 78, 170, 171
see also Phase II
Margarine, 20, 26, 66
McDonald's, 98–99
Meal basics, 21–38
beverages, 36–38
breakfast, 21–27
dessert, 34–35
dinner, 27–30, 31–34
lunch, 27–31
snacks, 35–36
Meal planning, 63–67
freezing meal-sized portions and, 67
importance of planning ahead and, 63–64
transforming your standbys into green-light recipes and, 65–67
Measurements:
changes in, at different rate than changes in weight, 130, 132
as predictor of state of your health, 41
recording each week, 50–51
waist-to-hip ratio and, 154
Meat, red, 8, 9, 67
filling your plate and, 20–21
G.I. Diet Food Guide for, 296–97
minimizing saturated fat in, 32
recipes for, 257–63
in restaurants, 96
serving size for, 20
Meatless main dishes, recipes for, 227–36
Menopause, 131, 132
Menstruation, 130
Metabolism, 19, 111, 131, 194
Milk, skim, 26, 37, 94
Minerals, 3
Mini-goals, 56
Molasses, 66
Monounsaturated fats, 7–8, 9, 151
Monthly e-letters, 198–99
Motivation for weight loss, 51–55
appearance and, 53
"before" photographs and, 138
clothing and, 53, 138, 139
energy level and, 53–54, 139
health improvements and, 54, 139
maintaining, 137–43
"shopping bag cure" and, 139–40
support from friends and family and, 140–42
$10 cure and, 142–43
Mountain biking, 174–75
Muscle, 41
body mass index (BMI) and, 18
energy burned by, 177
exercise and, 170, 171, 172, 176–77

N

National Academy of Sciences, 45
National Weight Control Registry, 170
Native Indians of Canada, 151–52

Nervousness. *See* Anxiety
Nutrition bars, 35, 94
Nuts, 9, 94, 197
  serving size for, 20
  as snack, 35

O

Oats and oatmeal, 4, 5, 25, 66, 94
Obesity, 77, 80
  body mass index (BMI) and, 18
  diabetes and, 151
  heart disease and stroke and, 150
  surge in rate of, 2
Oils:
  with "bad" and "really ugly" fats, 7
  best choices for, 66
  G.I. Diet Food Guide for, 294
  in G.I. Diet Clinic pantry, 47
  with "good" and "best" fats, 7–8
  green-light, serving size for, 20
Olive oil, 8, 20, 66
Olives, 8, 20, 197
Omega-3s, 8, 33
Orange juice, 36, 38
Osteoporosis, exercise and, 170
Outdoor activities, as exercise, 173–75
Overweight:
  body mass index (BMI) and, 18
  health risks associated with, 149–54
  societal biases and, 186
  surge in rate of, 2, 4

P

Palm oil, 7
Pancreas, 12
Pantry, G.I. Diet Clinic, 46–47
Partially hydrogenated oils, 7, 44
Pasta, 12, 34
  filling your plate and, 20–21
  G.I. Diet Food Guide for, 297
  in G.I. Diet Clinic pantry, 47
  in Phase II, 197
  serving size for, 20
Pasta sauces, G.I. Diet Food Guide for, 297
Peanut butter, 6, 87–88
Personality, weight loss and, 185–86
Phase I, 15, 18–38
  beverages in, 36–38
  breakfast in, 21–27
  combination of green-light protein, fats, and carbohydrates in, 20–21
  continuing with, until reaching target weight, 193
  determining whether to begin with, 15, 18
  dinner in, 27–30, 31–34
  lunch in, 27–31
  serving sizes in, 19–20
  snacks in, 19, 21, 35–36
  when to eat in, 18–19, 21
Phase II, xii, 15, 193–99
  alcohol in, 195–96
  breakfast in, 196
  chocolate in, 195, 196, 197
  dinner in, 197
  lunch in, 197
  serving sizes in, 193, 194–95
  snacks in, 197
  yellow-light foods in, xi, 193, 194, 196, 197
Photographs, motivation for weight loss and, 138
Pilates, 177–78
Pizza, 97
Planning ahead:
  importance of, 63–64
  traveling and, 94
  see also Meal planning
Plaque, 151
Plateaus, 111, 129–32
  changes in measurements and, 130, 132
Plates:
  "cleaning," 78–79, 118–19
  size of, 79
Polyunsaturated fats, 7, 8, 9, 151
Pork:
  Canadian bacon, 27, 196
  low-fat cuts of, 32
Portion sizes. *See* Serving sizes
Potatoes, 3, 13–14, 34, 96
  filling your plate and, 20–21
  in Phase II, 197
  serving size for, 20

Poultry, 9, 32, 67
filling your plate and, 20–21
G.I. Diet Food Guide for, 296–97
recipes for, 210, 224, 245–56
in restaurants, 96
serving size for, 20
Preliminary Phase, 15, 18–38
beverages in, 36–38
breakfast in, 21–27
combination of green-light protein, fats, and carbohydrates in, 20–21
determining whether to begin with, 15, 18
dinner in, 27–30, 31–34
lunch in, 27–31
serving sizes in, 19–20
snacks in, 19, 21, 35–36
when to eat in, 18–19, 21
Preserves, G.I. Diet Food Guide for, 299
Processed foods, 4–5, 14
Prostate cancer, 7, 152
Protein, 3, 8–9
adapting your standby recipes and, 67
animal sources of, 8, 32–33
boosting, 67
for breakfast, red-, yellow-, and green-light choices (charts), 22
digestive process and, 8, 9, 67
at dinner, 32–34
filling your plate and, 20–21
for lunch and dinner, red-, yellow-, and green-light choices (charts), 27–28
serving size for, 32
in snacks, 35
vegetable sources of, 8–9, 33–34

Q

Quiznos, 101–2

R

Red-light foods, xi, 13
replacing with green-light alternatives, 66, 119
$10 cure and, 142–43, 194
using in very limited quantities, 66
Resistance training, 171–72, 176–77
Restaurants, 93–104
see also Eating out; Fast food
Rewards:
for changing eating behaviors, 119
for exercise, food as, 78
for reaching mini-goals, 56
Rice, 14, 34, 96
filling your plate and, 20–21
serving size for, 20
Rowing machines, 176
Rubber exercise bands, 177
Running, 170, 173–74

S

Sadness, emotional eating and, 118, 120
Salads, 67
dining out and, 95, 96
holiday dinners and, 161
for lunch, 31
recipes for, 215–26
Salmon, 33
Salt, food labels and, 44–45
Sandwiches, 31
Satiety:
fats and, 6
fiber and, 5
low-G.I. carbohydrates and, 13, 14
protein and, 9
Saturated fats, 7, 9, 26, 66, 151
in red meat, minimizing, 32
Sauces, in restaurants, 96
Seafood. *See* Fish and seafood
Seasonality, weight loss and, 130
Seasonings, G.I. Diet Food Guide for, 292–93
Sedentary lifestyle, 2
Self-esteem:
boosted by weight loss, 53, 123
low, 118
Seltzer, 37
Serving sizes:
cleaning your plate and, 78–79, 118–19
eating out and, 93–94, 96
filling your plate and, 20–21
food labels and, 43
for green-light foods, 19–20
in Phase II, 193, 194–95
too-large, eating, 120

Setbacks, dealing with, 85–88
Sex, 170
Sexual abuse, 186
Shopping, 43–45
on empty stomach, 42–43, 79
and grocery lists for each week of G.I. Diet Clinic, 43, 64. *See also specific weeks*
label reading and, 43–45
planning ahead and, 43, 64, 65
"Shopping bag cure," 139–40
Shrimp, 33
Skeletal frame, 41
Ski machines, 176
Skim milk, 26, 37, 94
Skipping snacks or meals, 74, 109
breakfast and, 8, 75
Slip-ups, dealing with, 85–88
Smoking, 150
Snacks, 5, 35–36, 67, 76
cocktail parties and, 160
getting through hardest part of day and, 87
G.I. Diet Food Guide for, 298
in G.I. Diet Clinic pantry, 47
in Phase II, 197
in Preliminary Phase and Phase I, 19, 21
recipes for, 264–71
red-, yellow-, and green-light foods for (charts), 35–36
skipping, 74, 109
traveling and, 94
TV watching and, 119, 120
Social activities, eating during, 120
Social factors, weight-loss experience influenced by, 183–88
Sodium, food labels and, 44–45
Soft drinks, 36, 37, 78
Soluble fiber, 5, 66
Soups:
bean, 33
dining out and, 95–96
G.I. Diet Food Guide for, 299
holiday dinners and, 161
recipes for, 211–214
red-, yellow-, and green-light (charts), 30
Soy products, 8–9
Special events, 159–63
birthdays, 96, 102
cocktail parties, 160, 195–96
see also Holidays
Spices, 47
Splenda, 66–67
Sports, 175
Spreads:
G.I. Diet Food Guide for, 299
for sandwiches, 31
Squid, 33
Stadium food, 102
Stair climbers, 176
Starches, 3, 14
Steaks, 32, 197
Strength training, 171–72, 176–77
Stress, 137
emotional eating and, 118, 120
Stretching, 172
Stroke:
exercise and, 170
red wine and, 195
risk factors for, 7, 41, 44, 54, 149–51, 154
Substitute activities, 120–21
Subway (fast-food chain), 98
Sucralose (Splenda), 66–67
Sucrose, 44
Sugar:
adapting your standby recipes and, 66–67
food labels and, 44
G.I. Diet Food Guide for, 299
see also Blood sugar
"Sugar-free" snacks and desserts, 35
Sugar substitutes, 66–67
Sunflower oil, 7
Support from friends and family, 140–42
Sweeteners:
adapting your standby recipes and, 66–67
food labels and, 44
G.I. Diet Food Guide for, 299
sugar substitutes, 66–67
Sweet potatoes, 34, 161–62
Swimming, 171

T

Taco Bell, 100
Tai chi, 178

Target weight:
making it to, 193
reminding yourself of, 50, 137–38
setting, 40–42
Teas, 24, 37–38
herbal, 24, 38, 78
Tempura, 96
$10 cure, 142–43, 194
Textured vegetable protein (TVP), 33–34
"Thrift gene," 152
Time:
eating slowly vs. quickly and, 77, 95, 120
needed to prepare meals properly, 75–76
Tiredness, emotional eating and, 120
Toast, 25
Tofu, 9, 33
filling your plate and, 20–21
G.I. Diet Food Guide for, 296–97
Trans fats, 7, 44
Traveling, eating out while, 94
Treadmills, 176
Treats, high-sugar, high-fat, 79–80
Turkey, 32, 161
TV, snacking and, 119, 120

U

Unconscious eating, 77, 120–21
Unrealistic expectations, 119
about rate of weight loss, 109–12
Unsaturated fats, 7–8

V

Veal, low-fat cuts of, 32
Vegetable juices, 36
Vegetable oils:
with "bad" and "really ugly" fats, 7
best choices for, 66
in G.I. Diet Clinic pantry, 47
with "good" and "best" fats, 7–8
Vegetable oil spray, 32
Vegetables, 3, 5, 12
blood pressure and, 150–51
cooking, G.I. rating and, 14
in dinner, 34
filling your plate and, 20–21
G.I. Diet Food Guide for, 299–300
in G.I. Diet Clinic pantry, 46
holiday dinners and, 161
Vinegars, 47
Vitamins, 3, 14

W

Waist measurements:
as predictor of state of your health, 41
recording each week, 50–51
waist-to-hip ratio and, 154
Walking, 78, 170, 171, 173, 174
treadmills and, 176
Walnuts, 8
Warming up, 172
Water, 37, 95
not drinking enough, 77–78
Water retention, 44
estrogen and, 130, 131
menopause and, 131
Week 1, 50–62
diary for, 59
goals and rewards, 56
grocery list for, 62
nervousness about starting diet in, 55–56
optional meal plan for, 60–61
reasons for losing weight, 51–55
withdrawal symptoms in, 56–58
Week 2, 63–72
diary for, 68–69
grocery list for, 72
optional meal plan for, 70–71
topic: meal planning, 63–67
Week 3, 73–84
diary for, 81
grocery list for, 84
optional meal plan for, 82–83
topic: behavior change, 73–80
Week 4, 85–92
diary for, 89
grocery list for, 92
optional meal plan for, 90–91
topic: falling off the wagon, 85–88
Week 5, 93–108
diary for, 105
grocery list for, 108
optional meal plan for, 106–7

topic: eating out, 93–104
Week 6, 109–16
diary for, 112–13
grocery list for, 116
optional meal plan for, 114–15
topic: unrealistic expectations, 109–12
Week 7, 117–28
diary for, 124–25
grocery list for, 128
optional meal plan for, 126–27
topic: emotional eating, 117–23
Week 8, 129–36
diary for, 133
grocery list for, 136
optional meal plan for, 134–35
topic: reaching a plateau, 129–32
Week 9, 137–48
diary for, 144–45
grocery list for, 148
optional meal plan for, 146–47
topic: staying motivated, 137–43
Week 10, 149–58
diary for, 155
grocery list for, 158
optional meal plan for, 156–57
topic: health risks, 149–54
Week 11, 159–68
diary for, 164–65
grocery list for, 168
optional meal plan for, 166–67
topic: holidays, celebrations, and special events, 159–63
Week 12, 169–82
diary for, 179
grocery list for, 182
optional meal plan for, 180–81
topic: exercise, 169–78
Week 13, 183–92
diary for, 188–89
grocery list for, 192
optional meal plan for, 190–91
topic: when weight loss causes anxiety, 183–88
Week 13, beyond, 193–99
see also Phase II
Weight:
frequency of weigh-ins and, 130, 132
recording each week, 50–51
target. *See* Target weight
Weight loss:
average weekly rate of, 41, 109, 111
exercise and, 78, 170–71
fat consumption and, 6–7
low-G.I. foods and, 11, 12, 14
motivation for, 51–55. *See also* Motivations for weight loss
plateaus and, 111, 129–32
setting target for, 40–42. *See also* Target weight
"shopping bag cure" and, 139–40
slow and steady approach to, 109
social factors and, 183–88
unrealistic expectations about rate of, 109–12
Weight training, 171–72, 176–77
Wendy's, 100
When to eat, 21
White flour, 5
Whole grains, 5, 25, 66
Wine, 66, 195
Withdrawal symptoms, 56–58

Y

Yellow-light foods, xi, 13
in Phase II, xi, 193, 194, 196, 197
replacing with green-light alternatives, 66
using in very limited quantities, 66
Yoga, 178
Yogurt, 44
fat-free, 26

Recipe Index

A

Accompaniments:
- apple compote, 260–61
- mandarin salsa, 242–43
- *see also* Sauces

Almonds:
- creamy lemon squares, 279
- homemade muesli, 203
- homey oatmeal, 202
- orange chicken with, 250–51
- plum crumble, 275–76

Apple:
- berry crumble, 274
- bran muffins, 264–65
- chicken curry, 247
- compote, 260–61
- pie cookies, 278
- raspberry coffee cake, 272–73
- Waldorf chicken and rice salad, 226

Apricots, dried, in whole wheat fruit scones, 269

Argentinean flavors, in grilled tuna with *chimichurri* sauce, 241–42

Asian flavors:
- cold noodle salad with cucumber and sesame, 223
- fried rice with chicken, 246–47
- ginger-wasabi halibut, 240
- orange chicken with almonds, 250–51
- Thai red curry shrimp pasta, 244

Asparagus, in fettuccine primavera, 227–28

B

Barbecued chicken, zesty, 252–53

Barbecue sauce, zesty, 253

Barley risotto with leeks, lemon, and peas, 236

Beans and legumes:
- basic G.I. salad with, 216
- bean and onion pizza, 234–35
- beef and eggplant chili, 257
- chicken jambalaya, 256
- lentil and ham soup, 214
- minestrone, 212–13
- mixed bean salad, 222
- pecan brownies, 280–81
- Tuscan white bean soup, 213
- *see also* Chickpeas

Bean sprouts, in fried rice with chicken, 246–47

Beef:
- and eggplant chili, 257
- horseradish burgers, 258–59
- meat loaf, 259

Berry(ies):
- crumble, 274
- *see also* Cranberry(ies); Strawberry(ies)

Blackberries, in berry crumble, 274

Blueberries, in berry crumble, 274

Bran:
- apple muffins, 264–65
- apple raspberry coffee cake, 272–73
- carrot muffins, 267–68
- cranberry cinnamon muffins, 266–67
- creamy lemon squares, 279
- oat, in homemade muesli, 203
- vegetable crumble, 230–31

Bread(s):
- bean and onion pizza, 234–35
- Caesar salad, 216–17
- cinnamon French toast, 204
- strawberry tea, 270–71
- whole wheat fruit scones, 269
- *see also* Muffins

Breakfast, 202–10
- basic G.I., 215–16
- Canadian bacon omelet, 207
- cinnamon French toast, 204
- Italian omelet, 208

mini puffs, 206
muesli, homemade, 203
oatmeal, homey, 202
oatmeal buttermilk pancakes, 205
vegetarian omelet, 209
Western omelet, 210
Broccoli:
mini breakfast puffs, 206
salmon pasta, 238
vegetarian omelet, 209
Brownies, pecan, 280–81
Bulgur, in tabbouleh salad, 221
Burgers, horseradish, 258–59
Buttermilk oatmeal pancakes, 205

C

Cabbage, in tangy red and green coleslaw, 219
Caesar salad, 216–17
Cajun chicken jambalaya, 256
Cakes:
chocolate, one-bowl, 276–77
coffee, apple raspberry, 272–73
ganache icing for, 277
Canadian bacon:
minestrone, 212–13
omelet, 207
Western omelet, 210
Cannellini, in Tuscan white bean soup, 213
Carrot(s):
basic G.I. salad, 215–16
chicken curry, 247
fettuccine primavera, 227–28
minestrone, 212–13
muffins, 267–68
tangy red and green coleslaw, 219
vegetable crumble, 230–31
Celery:
chicken curry, 247
Waldorf chicken and rice salad, 226
Cheddar cheese, low-fat:
vegetable crumble, 230–31
vegetarian omelet, 209
Cheese:
sauce, 232–33
see also Cottage cheese, fat-free; Feta cheese, light; Mozzarella cheese, part-skim
Chicken, 245–56
basic G.I. salad with, 216
curry, 247
fried rice with, 246–47
jambalaya, 256
noodle soup, quick and easy, 211
orange, with almonds, 250–51
pasta salad, G.I., 224
and rice Waldorf salad, 226
rigatoni with mini meatballs, 254–55
schnitzel, 248–49
spicy roast, with tomatoes and tarragon, 249–50
tarragon with mushrooms, 245
zesty barbecued, 252–53
Chickpeas (garbanzo beans):
basic G.I. salad with, 216
crab salad in tomato shells, 225
crunchy, 271
fried rice with chicken, 246–47
minestrone, 212–13
mixed bean salad, 222
tabbouleh salad, 221
vegetarian moussaka, 232–33
Chili, beef and eggplant, 257
Chinese flavors:
fried rice with chicken, 246–47
orange chicken with almonds, 250–51
Chocolate:
cake, one-bowl, 276–77
ganache icing, 277
Cilantro, in *chimichurri* sauce, 241
Cinnamon:
cranberry bran muffins, 266–67
French toast, 204
Citrus-poached haddock, 239
Coffee cake, apple raspberry, 272–73
Cold noodle salad with cucumber and sesame, 223
Coleslaw, tangy red and green, 219
Compote, apple, 260–61
Cookies, apple pie, 278
Cottage cheese, fat-free:
easy-bake lasagna, 228–29
vegetarian moussaka, 232–33
Crab salad in tomato shells, 225

Cranberry(ies):
cinnamon bran muffins, 266–67
dried, in whole wheat fruit scones, 269
Creamy lemon squares, 279
Crumbles:
berry, 274
plum, 275–76
vegetable, 230–31
Crunchy chickpeas, 271
Cucumber:
basic G.I. salad, 215–16
cold noodle salad with sesame and, 223
Greek salad, 218
mandarin salsa, 242–43
mixed bean salad, 222
raita salad, 220
Curry:
chicken, 247
Thai red, shrimp pasta, 244

D

Desserts, 272–81
apple pie cookies, 278
apple raspberry coffee cake, 272–73
berry crumble, 274
chocolate cake, one-bowl, 276–77
lemon squares, creamy, 279
pecan brownies, 280–81
plum crumble, 275–76
strawberry tea bread with sliced berries, 270–71
Dijon pork medallions, 261–62

E

Egg, liquid:
Canadian bacon omelet, 207
cinnamon French toast, 204
Italian omelet, 208
mini breakfast puffs, 206
vegetarian omelet, 209
Western omelet, 210
Eggplant:
and beef chili, 257
rigatoni with mini meatballs, 254–55
vegetarian moussaka, 232–33

F

Feta cheese, light:
bean and onion pizza, 234–35
Greek salad, 218
mini breakfast puffs, 206
vegetarian moussaka, 232–33
Fettuccine primavera, 227–28
Fish and seafood, 237–44
crab salad in tomato shells, 225
fish fillet, G.I., 237
haddock, citrus-poached, 239
halibut, ginger-wasabi, 240
salmon pasta, 238
shrimp pasta, Thai red curry, 244
tuna, grilled, with *chimichurri* sauce, 241–42
whitefish, pan-seared, with mandarin salsa, 242–43
French toast, cinnamon, 204
Fried rice with chicken, 246–47
Fruit scones, whole wheat, 269

G

Ganache icing, 277
Garbanzo beans. *See* Chickeas
Garlic, in *chimichurri* sauce, 241
Ginger-wasabi halibut, 240
Greek (flavors):
salad, 218
vegetarian moussaka, 232–33
Grilled tuna with *chimichurri* sauce, 241–42

H

Haddock, citrus-poached, 239
Halibut, ginger-wasabi, 240
Ham:
and lentil soup, 214
Western omelet, 210
Horseradish burgers, 258–59

I

Icing, ganache, 277
Indian flavors:
chicken curry, 247
raita salad, 220

Italian flavors:
barley risotto with leeks, lemon, and peas, 236
bean and onion pizza, 234–35
easy-bake lasagna, 228–29
fettuccine primavera, 227–28
minestrone, 212–13
omelet, 208
rigatoni with mini meatballs, 254–55
salmon pasta, 238
Tuscan white bean soup, 213

J

Jambalaya, chicken, 256

K

Kale, in Tuscan white bean soup, 213
Kidney beans:
basic G.I. salad with, 216
bean and onion pizza, 234–35
beef and eggplant chili, 257
chicken jambalaya, 256
minestrone, 212–13
mixed bean salad, 222

L

Lasagna, easy-bake, 228–29
Leeks:
barley risotto with lemon, peas and, 236
vegetable crumble, 230–31
Lemon:
barley risotto with leeks, peas and, 236
squares, creamy, 279
Lentil and ham soup, 214
Lettuce:
basic G.I. salad, 215–16
iceberg, in Greek salad, 218
romaine, in Caesar salad, 216–17

M

Main dishes, 227–63
barley risotto with leeks, lemon, and peas, 236
bean and onion pizza, 234–35
beef and eggplant chili, 257
burgers, horseradish, 258–59
chicken, orange, with almonds, 250–51
chicken, spicy roast, with tomatoes and tarragon, 249–50
chicken, zesty barbecued, 252–53
chicken curry, 247
chicken jambalaya, 256
chicken schnitzel, 248–49
chicken tarragon with mushrooms, 245
fettuccine primavera, 227–28
fish fillet, G.I., 237
fried rice with chicken, 246–47
haddock, citrus-poached, 239
halibut, ginger-wasabi, 240
lasagna, easy-bake, 228–29
meat loaf, 259
pork chops, mushroom gravy, 263
pork medallions Dijon, 261–62
pork tenderloin with apple compote, 260–61
rigatoni with mini meatballs, 254–55
salmon pasta, 238
shrimp pasta, Thai red curry, 244
tuna, grilled, with *chimichurri* sauce, 241–42
vegetable crumble, 230–31
vegetarian moussaka, 232–33
whitefish, pan-seared, with mandarin salsa, 242–43
Mandarin salsa, 242–43
Meat, 257–63
basic G.I. salad with, 216
beef and eggplant chili, 257
burgers, horseradish, 258–59
loaf, 259
pork chops, mushroom gravy, 263
pork medallions Dijon, 261–62
pork tenderloin with apple compote, 260–61
Meatballs, mini, rigatoni with, 254–55
Meatless main dishes, 227–36
barley risotto with leeks, lemon, and peas, 236
bean and onion pizza, 234–35
fettuccine primavera, 227–28
lasagna, easy-bake, 228–29
vegetable crumble, 230–31
vegetarian moussaka, 232–33

Middle Eastern tabbouleh salad, 221
Minestrone, 212–13
Mini breakfast puffs, 206
Mint, in tabbouleh salad, 221
Mixed bean salad, 222
Moussaka, vegetarian, 232–33
Mozzarella cheese, part-skim:
  easy-bake lasagna, 228–29
  Italian omelet, 208
Muesli, homemade, 203
Muffins:
  apple bran, 264–65
  carrot, 267–68
  cranberry cinnamon bran, 266–67
Mushroom(s):
  chicken tarragon with, 245
  easy-bake lasagna, 228–29
  fried rice with chicken, 246–47
  gravy pork chops, 263
  Italian omelet, 208
  vegetable crumble, 230–31
  vegetarian omelet, 209

N

Noodle(s):
  chicken, soup, quick and easy, 211
  salad, cold, with cucumber and sesame, 223
  see also Pasta

O

Oat(meal)(s):
  apple pie cookies, 278
  berry crumble, 274
  bran, in homemade muesli, 203
  buttermilk pancakes, 205
  homemade muesli, 203
  homey, 202
  plum crumble, 275–76
Omelets:
  Canadian bacon, 207
  Italian, 208
  vegetarian, 209
Onion and bean pizza, 234–35
Orange:
  chicken with almonds, 250–51
  mandarin salsa, 242–43

P

Pancakes, oatmeal buttermilk, 205
Parsley:
  chimichurri sauce, 241
  tabbouleh salad, 221
Pasta:
  cold noodle salad with cucumber and sesame, 223
  fettuccine primavera, 227–28
  lasagna, easy-bake, 228–29
  minestrone, 212–13
  rigatoni with mini meatballs, 254–55
  salad, G.I., 224
  salmon, 238
  Thai red curry shrimp, 244
  whole wheat, in mixed bean salad, 222
Peas:
  barley risotto with leeks, lemon and, 236
  fettuccine primavera, 227–28
Pecan(s):
  apple raspberry coffee cake, 272–73
  berry crumble, 274
  brownies, 280–81
  plum crumble, 275–76
Peppers:
  basic G.I. salad, 215–16
  beef and eggplant chili, 257
  chicken jambalaya, 256
  easy-bake lasagna, 228–29
  fettuccine primavera, 227–28
  mandarin salsa, 242–43
  mini breakfast puffs, 206
  vegetable crumble, 230–31
  vegetarian moussaka, 232–33
  vegetarian omelet, 209
  Western omelet, 210
Pizza, bean and onion, 234–35
Plum crumble, 275–76
Pork:
  chops, mushroom gravy, 263
  medallions Dijon, 261–62
  tenderloin with apple compote, 260–61
  see also Canadian bacon; Ham

R

Raita salad, 220

Raspberry(ies):
apple coffee cake, 272–73
berry crumble, 274
Red curry shrimp pasta, Thai, 244
Rice:
chicken curry, 247
chicken jambalaya, 256
and chicken Waldorf salad, 226
fried, with chicken, 246–47
Rigatoni with mini meatballs, 254–55
Risotti, barley, with leeks, lemon, and peas, 236
Romaine lettuce, in Caesar salad, 216–17

S

Salad dressings:
basic G.I. vinaigrette, 215–16
Caesar, 217
Salads, 215–26
basic G.I., 215–16
Caesar, 216–17
cold noodle, with cucumber and sesame, 223
crab, in tomato shells, 225
Greek, 218
mixed bean, 222
pasta, G.I., 224
raita, 220
tabbouleh, 221
tangy red and green coleslaw, 219
Waldorf chicken and rice, 226
Salmon:
basic G.I. salad with, 216
pasta, 238
Salsa, mandarin, 242–43
Sauces:
barbecue, zesty, 253
cheese, 232–33
chimichurri, 241
Sausage, chicken, in G.I. pasta salad, 224
Schnitzel, chicken, 248–49
Scones, whole wheat fruit, 269
Seafood. *See* Fish and seafood
Sesame (seeds):
cold noodle salad with cucumber and, 223
toasting, 223
vegetable crumble, 230–31
Shrimp pasta, Thai red curry, 244
Snacks, 264–71
apple bran muffins, 264–65
carrot muffins, 267–68
chickpeas, crunchy, 271
cranberry cinnamon bran muffins, 266–67
strawberry tea bread, 270–71
whole wheat fruit scones, 269
Soups, 211–14
chicken noodle, quick and easy, 211
ham and lentil, 214
minestrone, 212–13
white bean, Tuscan, 213
Spicy roast chicken with tomatoes and tarragon, 249–50
Spinach:
easy-bake lasagna, 228–29
minestrone, 212–13
raita salad, 220
Strawberry(ies):
berry crumble, 274
cinnamon French toast, 204
tea bread, 270–71
Sunflower seeds, in homemade muesli, 203
Sweet potatoes, in vegetable crumble, 230–31

T

Tabbouleh salad, 221
Tangy red and green coleslaw, 219
Tarragon:
chicken with mushrooms, 245
spicy roast chicken with tomatoes and, 249–50
Thai red curry shrimp pasta, 244
Tofu:
basic G.I. salad with, 216
easy-bake lasagna, 228–29
fettuccine primavera, 227–28
fried rice with, 247
Tomato(es):
basic G.I. salad, 215–16
chicken jambalaya, 256
fettuccine primavera, 227–28
Greek salad, 218
minestrone, 212–13
mixed bean salad, 222
raita salad, 220

rigatoni with mini meatballs, 254–55
shells, crab salad in, 225
spicy roast chicken with tarragon and, 249–50
tabbouleh salad, 221
vegetarian moussaka, 232–33
zesty barbecue sauce, 253
Tuna:
basic G.I. salad with, 216
grilled, with *chimichurri* sauce, 241–42
Turkey:
pasta salad, G.I., 224
rigatoni with mini meatballs, 254–55
Western omelet, 210
Tuscan white bean soup, 213

V

Vegetable crumble, 230–31
Vegetarian moussaka, 232–33
Vegetarian omelet, 209
Vinaigrette, basic G.I., 215–16

W

Waldorf chicken and rice salad, 226
Walnuts:
berry crumble, 274
Waldorf chicken and rice salad, 226
Wasabi-ginger halibut, 240
Western omelet, 210
Wheat germ:
homemade muesli, 203
homey oatmeal, 202
White bean soup, Tuscan, 213
Whitefish, pan-seared, with mandarin salsa, 242–43
Whole wheat fruit scones, 269

Y

Yogurt, low-fat, in raita salad, 220

Z

Zesty barbecued chicken, 252–53
Zucchini:
rigatoni with mini meatballs, 254–55
vegetable crumble, 230–31
yellow, in fettuccine primavera, 227–28